# REWIRING EXCELLENCE
## HARDWIRED TO REWIRED

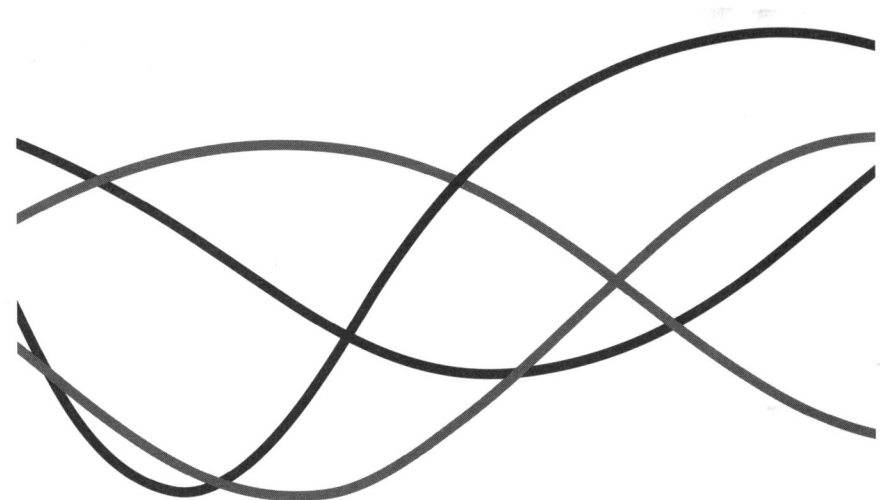

**QUINT STUDER**
WITH DAN COLLARD

Copyright © 2023 by Quint Studer and Dan Collard

All rights reserved.

Published by:
The Gratitude Group Publishing
350 West Cedar St., Suite 300
Pensacola, FL 32502
www.thegratitudegroup.com

ISBN: 978-1-7370789-3-7

Library of Congress Control Number: 2023944882

The stories in this book are true. However, some names and identifying details have been changed to protect the privacy of all concerned.

All rights reserved. No part of this book may be used or reproduced in any form or by any means, or stored in a database or retrieval system without the prior written permission of the publisher, except in the case of brief quotations embodied in critical articles or reviews. Making copies of any part of this book for any purpose other than your own personal use is a violation of United States copyright laws. Entering any of the contents into a computer for mailing list or database purposes is strictly prohibited unless written authorization is obtained from The Gratitude Group Publishing.

Printed in the United States of America

To all past, present, and future Fire Starters

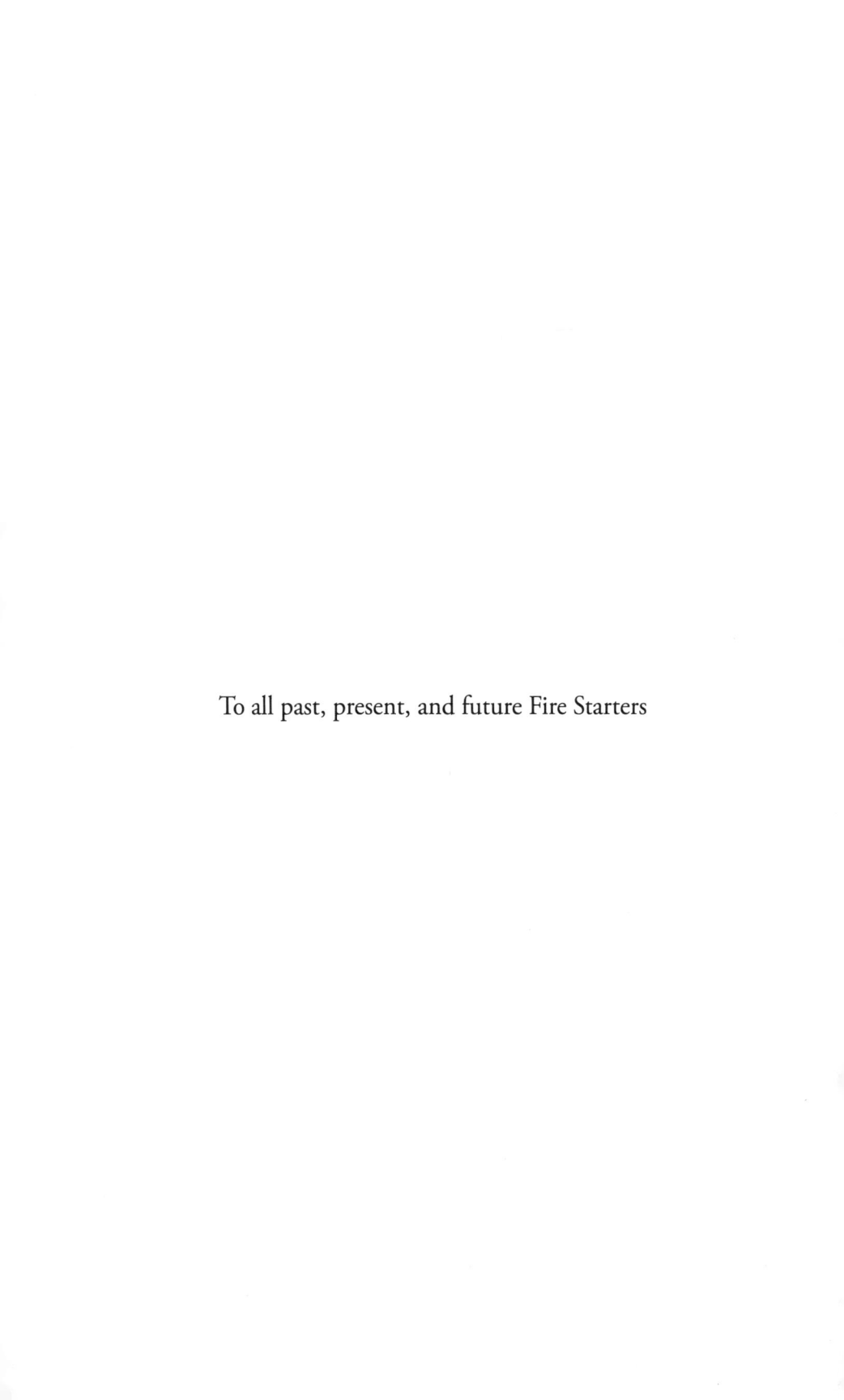

# Table of Contents

*Rewiring Excellence* Is a Living Book.................i

Preface....................................iii

Introduction: What Does It Mean to Rewire?...........v

Chapter 1: Diagnosing the Need to Rewire.............1

Chapter 2: Rewiring Organizational Assessments:
A Walk Through the Human Capital Ecosystem...........9

Chapter 3: Rewiring the Selection and Onboarding Processes...25

Chapter 4: Rewiring Patient and Employee Rounding....33

Chapter 5: Rewiring Leader Development..............45

Chapter 6: Rewiring Skill Building and the Evaluation Process..53

Chapter 7: Rewiring Physician Ownership.............61

Chapter 8: Rewiring Well-Being......................69

Chapter 9: Rewiring Retention.......................77

Chapter 10: Summary.................................83

Endnotes............................................87

About the Authors...................................89

About Healthcare Plus Solutions Group...............93

Other Books from Quint Studer.......................95

# *Rewiring Excellence* Is a Living Book

You might be wondering: Why is *Rewiring Excellence* available only online? The answer is that it's meant to be a living book. For starters, it's easier to access for readers. But the biggest reason is that it can be updated regularly.

We hope you will work with us as you discover tools and techniques that you find useful. We are all committed to making healthcare the best it can be. So, what works for you may help others.

We love printed books. A drawback is that by the time one is printed, six months to a year may have passed since the writing was completed. Things can change greatly from the completion of a manuscript to the publishing of a book. As we're out in the field each week, it is apparent that we are in an ever-changing world.

While we want to make this book available quickly and electronically, we do know some people prefer print, so we will do a short print run as well.

As we share with organizations the actions in the book and see the impact, we feel that timing is important. The actions in this book may help someone working in healthcare stay. I know they will help organizations navigate the choppy waters of our industry.

As you read the material, please let us know any questions you have, ideas you find that work, or suggestions that will make the book better. We are on this healthcare journey together.

Thank you.

# Preface

At first, you might have thought the title of this book had a typo. After all, since 2003, there has been a book that thousands of leaders have carried with them through their careers. It has become a mainstay in graduate courses in healthcare leadership. Its content has been cited in numerous articles. You might say it has been "hardwired" into our industry.

And yet...here we are today. It's a different world from 2003. It's a time that calls for different solutions...solutions that fit today versus 20 years ago. Medicine has evolved; technology has evolved. Wouldn't the way we solve healthcare's greatest challenges also evolve?

It's time to rewire. This does not mean certain actions don't remain hardwired. What it means is if an action is working, leave it alone. There are times when some aspects stay hardwired, yet components are rewired.

This is more than a book about changing times. It's a book that brings every bit of necessary passion to an industry that needs it now more than ever. It's a book of doable approaches for an industry where sometimes even the most straightforward ideas are at risk of being overcomplicated. And it is a book that I call a "living book." It will continue to be refined as we learn more.

Who best to turn to for breaking down complex ideas into bite-size chunks…and making them accomplishable? The industry's best friend and advocate for so many years, Quint Studer. If you're a veteran leader, you'll recognize Quint's approach to creating solutions. If you're a new leader, you'll appreciate his gift for making the daunting seem doable. If you're a student or an aspiring leader, get ready for a healthy dose of reality so you can enter the world of healthcare leadership with an eyes-wide-open view.

Get ready to rewire.

—Dan Collard

# Introduction: What Does It Mean to Rewire?

Over the years, I have made use of various mental health services. During times, fear gets ahold of me. Fear of letting people down. Fear of failure. Fear of death. During this journey, the need to rewire my thinking becomes clear. This means changing the pattern of thinking that triggered my fears. For example, learning to say, "I get to," instead of, "I have to," or, "I must," has made a difference. That single change makes the action itself feel better. Instead of saying, "I have to go on the road this week," now it's, "I get to go on the road and work with great people."

Another one of my habits is projecting failure or anticipating the worst possible outcome. My rationalization is, "If I can handle the worst, then I will be prepared for whatever happens." That's not a bad thing if a hurricane is coming. However, done on a regular basis, it is exhausting and physically and mentally damaging. Today when this happens, my response is to engage in positive self-talk. For example, for years before every presentation, my mind would go to, *This is the presentation that will go bad.* Now my thought process is, *I have done* so many of these and they have gone well, so this one will go well today. When we wake up and say to ourselves, *Today is going to be a great day*, we usually find that it is. Every morning, my practice is to text a group that includes three other people; we each share three things we are grateful for from the day before. These are all examples of how we can rewire our thoughts and our language.

The word "rewire" also seems to fit today's healthcare environment. When we used the word "hardwire" years ago, it made sense, and sometimes it still can be the best word to describe a process. It means to put tools and methods in place so they happen consistently. The downside is that as things evolve in healthcare, there are tools, techniques, and actions that are no longer working or that don't work as well as they initially did. Yet they keep being used because they are hardwired. The bottom line is that some things benefit from never being changed, while others need to be changed to account for new circumstances. This is where rewiring comes in.

When is rewiring needed? A good question to ask for all actions is, "How is it working?" If the desired results are achieved, leave it alone. If results are not there, then it is time to relook at the situation. I was watching a video of Steve Jobs recently. (It's so sad he is no longer with us physically.) He talked about being bold enough to make what you create obsolete. A natural barrier to doing so is denial: the insistence that it's still working even when the facts say differently.

We are so fortunate to be contacted by many individuals. They want to feel better, like they used to feel. We share that this is very possible. However, it means letting go of much of the past. When the first fax machine came out, it was exciting. Yet, few would want to go back to faxing. Think about the early mobile phones. They were heavy, and no one today would carry a heavy bag phone around given the

## INTRODUCTION: WHAT DOES IT MEAN TO REWIRE?

modern versions available. Yet moving forward is not always easy. People are afraid to let go.

Today, we must rewire many of the current methods. While it's great to have lots of steps in place to achieve optimal employee engagement, physician engagement, and patient experience, what if they are not doable? What if the facts show they are not working as we wish they were? What if the structure or the rigid nature of the steps takes away the authenticity? What if the person on the receiving end of a technique feels like part of a transaction versus feeling valued as part of a relationship?

At a recent talk, I shared that my goal is to make many of the tools and techniques recommended over the years obsolete. It is not because that's my wish; it is because I have learned better ways to achieve the outcomes. That means the newest tools and tactics, not obsolete ones. While speaking these words, Steve Jobs' message was ringing in my ears.

We are in a world of perpetual rewiring. Yes, some actions are best hardwired, as they continue to be valuable. For example, I have hardwired morning prayers and am very consistent with them. However, even with something as vital as prayers, they are rewired a bit at times as needed. Likewise, people have learned over the years to shake up their workouts, for the same actions every time will lose impact and ultimately won't yield outcomes.

The beauty of rewiring is that it often makes things more doable, more flexible, more enjoyable, and more likely to achieve better outcomes.

We look forward to sharing in this book several "rewire" examples that work, as well as a process to diagnose and design your own rewires.

Thank you for all you do to keep healthcare excellent as the industry and world evolve around us.

—Quint Studer

CHAPTER 1

# Diagnosing the Need to Rewire

Years ago, in searching for a term to describe putting in place a tool, action, or method that would stick, the word "hardwired" came to mind. I am sure I read it somewhere. The word reminded me of projects my father worked on. He was a mechanic and a handyman. In some situations, he would put in a steel pipe and run wires through it. This protected the wires from various elements that could damage them. The pipe also held the wires steady and in place.

How can an organization create consistency and sustain high performance? There are some actions that should be hardwired, meaning not adjusted. The wire going through the pipe demonstrated that some systems are built to not be flexible and thus very hard to change. This is a good technique when the external environment stays the same, the workforce is very consistent, technology has little or no adjustments, and the hardwired actions and tools are achieving the desired outcomes.

As mentioned earlier, the need to rewire does not mean that what was implemented was wrong or did not work at the time. If they didn't work, the tools, processes, and actions would not have been put in place. The key is being willing and able to rethink things when circumstances change.

*Bounce: The Art of Turning Tough Times into Triumph* was written by Keith McFarland in 2009. It is a great book on how companies can bounce back after a financial downturn. In looking at late 2008/early 2009, the financial meltdown was very serious. Fast-forward to more recently and after the pandemic, organizations are experiencing even more challenges as they try to bounce back. The pandemic increased the acceleration of telehealth. It also increased the number of people who can work virtually. In *Bounce*, McFarland stated that two emotions that keep an organization from moving forward with the urgency needed are denial and nostalgia—denial of the depth and scope of the situation and nostalgia to go back to what once was. Denial is not the issue with the intense challenges facing all in healthcare. Nostalgia does rear up at times.

We receive calls from CEOs and others. We are grateful that people reach out. Many say, "It feels like we should just get back to the basics." As part of diagnosing an organization whose performance isn't where they want it to be, we'll traditionally ask two questions: 1. "What if a leader (or group of leaders) wasn't here when the basics were introduced?" and 2. "What if the basics have changed?"

In diagnosing, it is important to see why what worked in the past seems to not be working as well (or at all) in the present. Is it the tools that were put in place? Is it the process? Is it the frontline staff? Is it leadership? What other factors have impacted the outcomes?

*Experience* is a big one. The number of resignations that have taken place due to the pandemic means there are many people who are new to their roles. Even without the pandemic, the aging of the population meant there were going to be more retirements than normal. The pandemic increased the number of departures. Now we're in what we call "the one-up world." People tend to be in a role one up from where they were. It is not unusual for more than 20 percent of people in a leadership role to have less than three years' experience leading. Then, there is another 20 percent of people who are experienced in leadership; however, they're now in a different leadership role.

Here is an example: We were at an organization that is very well respected. All those in a leadership position were attending an off-site session. The CEO led off the day sharing the number "1,185," asking the group what they thought it represented. People had fun guessing. The answer turned out to be the number of days since they had all been together in person in a system-wide leadership session. In working with the human resource department, we learned that 43 percent of those in attendance had not been at the session 1,185 days ago. Some were brand new to the organization. Some had gone from an hourly staff position to a leadership role. What this meant was 57 percent of the attendees had a recollection of what being a leader at the organization used to be like. The other 43 percent did not. Imagine being at an event where people are sharing what a great time they had four years ago. While fun to hear, there's a different perception for those who were not at the event. This is the reality for leaders who became leaders after March 2020: Many could end up feeling like they'll eternally be three years behind everyone else.

It could be that what worked in the past may not work as well now due to the experience level of the workforce, including those in leadership roles. In most instances when a person is new, it is understood it will take them time to gain the skills those with more experience have. Yet the (often unspoken) expectation is the person new in leadership will pick up where the person they replaced left off, with performance expectations and more. For example, a new manager is still expected to achieve the labor budget and so on. Our work with people new in leadership shows that skills like working with staff scheduling and financial tools are not easy to manage day one. It is not that the tools are not good; it just takes time. Items like training and development need to be rewired. There is more to come on that in the following chapters.

What are some specific things to diagnose? When it comes to patient experience and the measure often used for inpatient care (HCAHPS), the questions, methodology, etc. can be debated; however, it is national data, so it is comparing apples to apples. Even before the pandemic, patient perception of experience had been stagnant since 2016. This was not due to lack of passion, dedication, or resources. As a matter of fact, there are more resources focused on patient experience now than in the past. We can't blame the pandemic as the only reason for the stagnation as results had been flat prior to COVID. The question then is, "What are some explanations for the stagnation?"

Here are some observations.

Due to so much complexity, helping people understand the connection between patient experience and clinical outcomes may have lessened. Connecting patient experience to clinical outcomes connects to values. Once an action is linked to values in employees' minds, that action is more likely to be taken. In fact, it cannot *not* be taken. Our experience is that when the connection is made that a patient will have a better clinical outcome when listened to, when the facility is clean, when medications and treatment plans are understood and so forth, the patient and family rates the experience highly.

When patient experience measurement was relatively new, people thought it was more focused on hospitality. Hospitality is important. However, for healthcare professionals, connecting patient experience to clinical outcomes created a deeper understanding of experience. Due to the work of many, today very few people, if any, question the need for patient experience. However, due to so many new people, the connection to clinical outcomes may not be as understood as it needs to be. It is always a good time to reconnect experience to clinical outcomes.

Another factor is that our attempts to improve the patient experience have gotten too complex. Even the best intentions can have negative consequences. In 1993, at Holy Cross Hospital in Chicago, when we first experienced rounding to improve the patient experience, we learned from a nurse leader named Michelle Walsko. Her patient care area had better results than the other areas. We met with her to find out what she did differently. It turned out that she visited all the new admits, introduced herself, shared her card, and explained how to reach her. She assured the patient that everyone was committed to making sure they received very good care. She asked how things were. She mentioned items she wanted the patient to be aware of. She would write down things to remember on a note card, like people to recognize, or an item to follow up on, or a patient she wanted to follow up with. And her unit's patient experience was in the top percentiles.

Michelle was our benchmark. Her approach was scaled throughout the hospital. It was a great experience. There were lots of people to recognize, and, at times, there were items to follow up on or fix. It was inspiring.

Over the years, the one question Michelle asked became two and then more questions—all with good intentions. Today nurse managers might be tasked with asking from 5 to 11 questions. The record is 17 questions expected to be asked. The note card or census sheet became an iPad. At times, there was more than one tool to use in documentation. What started out as a few actions meant to build relationships slowly moved into a process that can feel like a transaction. Now the inpatient rounding practice on new admits has moved to all patients every day. "Did you receive very good care?" and "How are we doing?" kept growing. The approach of "more questions and more patients" has at times led to worse, not better, outcomes.

In meeting with a nurse manager, I asked her how many patients are usually on the unit. The answer was 42. We then asked how many patients she was expected to see each day. The answer was all of them. And she was expected to document them all in a software tool. I asked her, "What are the chances that you will ask 210 questions?" She shared that it could not happen. We figured if she spent three minutes with each patient, it would take two hours (and that included no follow-up). The nurse manager felt trapped in some ways. Does she tell her leader she cannot do it? How does she fill out the software program?

This is a perfect opportunity to rewire the rounding. There is more to come on that later. The point is that tools that sound nice and that may work in a perfect healthcare world may not always work in reality. With the increase in questions, what could be doable has often become undoable.

Another example is key words at key times. Choosing the right words can be an incredibly powerful way to shape the patient experience. However, in our enthusiasm to become better and better, it is possible to take a tactic and make it too complicated. Healthcare people are authentic. Checklists and scripting can take away from authenticity and feeling valued.

## DIAGNOSING THE NEED TO REWIRE

In 1995, my youngest son was in an accident during a family camping trip. He ended up in an intensive care unit in a hospital in Rapid City. Today he is fine. However, during the first 48-72 hours after the accident, we were on edge, wondering if our son would live. We were in a city we had never been in, at an unfamiliar hospital. Of course, as anyone would, we wanted our son to be in a place where he could receive great care. Was this it?

In speaking with the physician in the intensive care unit, in my nervousness, I asked him where he went to medical school. He replied, "the University of Michigan." He went on to say that he stayed to do a residency in pediatrics and a fellowship in critical care, and he was boarded in both pediatrics and critical care medicine. He then offered that he grew up in Rapid City and always wanted to come back home. I went back into my son's room and said to my wife, Rishy, "We are fortunate to be in this hospital." We were still worried about our son's condition but no longer that he was in the wrong place. This led me to think about how words have the power to reduce or increase anxiety.

When I was with Studer Group®, we were working with a large system that wanted to scale "key words." This is where the acronym AIDET® was born. It stands for **A**cknowledge the patient, **I**ntroduce self and experience, share how long things will take (**D**uration), give an **E**xplanation or narrate the care or process, and say **T**hank you.[1] The acronym was meant as a clue to help people remember, which is a good thing. However, the intent can be misunderstood. AIDET was not intended to "always include all five letters and always in that order." What was meant to be a tactic for reducing patient anxiety can become another "transactional" encounter that feels scripted. When that happens, it does not seem natural, and the care provider feels they are not trusted. This is another opportunity to look at rewiring.

If you're wondering if a tool or tactic needs rewiring, the questions to ask are: *Is the current system achieving the needed results? Is what is currently being asked doable? Does what's being done feel authentic? Do these actions build relationships?* If you are not sure the answer is yes, it is time to examine them more closely.

There are many more items to take a fresh look at. Let's move on to some rewiring recommendations.

CHAPTER 2

# Rewiring Organizational Assessments: A Walk Through the Human Capital Ecosystem

Organizations must look outward and inward. Much of the strategic planning has happened in response to or anticipation of external forces and/or competition.

For example, a SWOT analysis (*Strengths, Weaknesses, Opportunities,* and *Threats*) is a good method. This analysis typically covers most of the elements across a balanced scorecard to solidify or fine tune the strategy. SWOTs are always a good opportunity to hold up the mirror organizationally, especially as it relates to the external environment.

As we emerged from the pandemic, we found ourselves facing stronger headwinds than ever before in areas like staffing (both sides of the equation: attracting and retaining talent), a decline in engagement (which paralleled trust in leadership), and an even more apparent lack of utilization of well-being resources. We realized that what we were facing wasn't a constellation of isolated issues but was more of a holistic problem, with one element impacting many others. By the same token, we knew that if we could strengthen any of the elements, they would, in turn, strengthen the others.

Thus, we realized there was an opportunity to reimagine and rewire the environment connected *internally* to an organization's people element. We call it the Human Capital Ecosystem™. An "ecosystem," of course, is a network of many interdependent elements within the organization. Like an ecosystem in nature, these interconnecting components are linked together. They interact with each other and with their environment to create outcomes—in the case of the Human Capital Ecosystem, an organization filled with fully engaged individuals who have a strong sense of belonging. This framework is designed to help organizations focus on how they attract, retain, and engage talent.

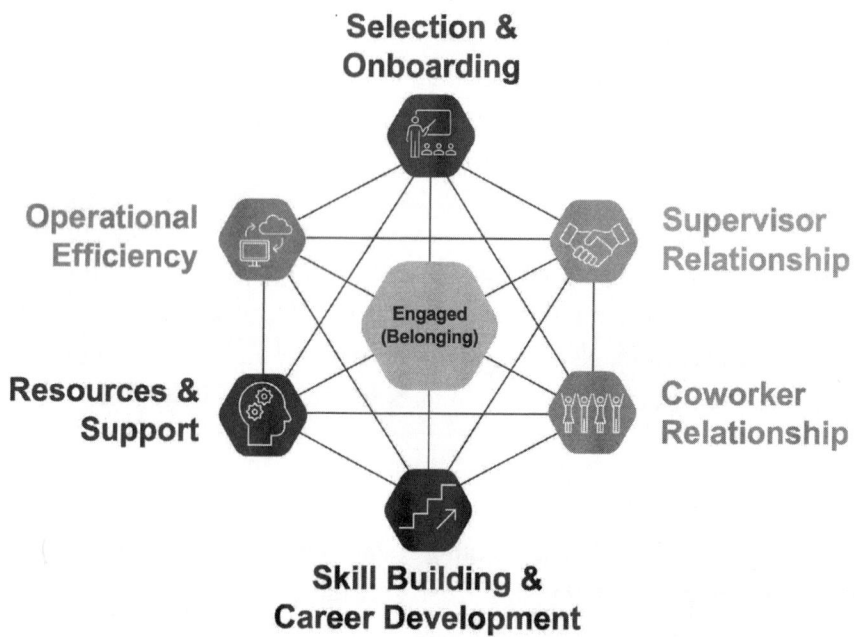

This is a leader-friendly version of holding up the mirror to look at how we've done things in the past and how we might reimagine things going forward. What's in? What's out? This process gives the organization the opportunity to ask for and listen to the voice of the entire leadership team and more. As you'll see referenced later in the explanation of each of the ecosystem elements, engaging the all-important middle leader group is key to building (or, in some cases, rebuilding) trust. If senior teams do a good job of saying "we want your input" and then acting upon the results, middle leaders will quickly align and carry important messages across their departments.

## How the Human Capital Ecosystem Assessment Works

We ask two questions per ecosystem component, typically engaging the entire leadership team of an organization. (We'll describe the process below, but for now, let's focus on the questions themselves.)

For **Selection and Onboarding**, we ask:

1. How would you rate the employee selection process? (Prescribed candidate profile, screening and interviewing process used consistently.)

2. How effective is [insert Organization Name] in making the employee onboarding an effective talent strategy? (Continuous process that minimizes turnover and improves employee engagement.)

For **Supervisor Relationship**, we ask:

1. How would middle managers rate the support they receive from senior leadership? (While we are using the term "middle

managers" here, we also use "middle leaders" in this book. The two are interchangeable.)

2. How well do you feel information is cascaded from the senior leadership team to frontline employees?

For **Coworker Relationship**, we ask:

1. How well do you feel employees at [insert Organization Name] live the Standards of Behavior?

2. How would you rate relationships between departments?

For **Skill Building and Career Development**, we ask:

1. How well is the current system of training and development providing leaders with the needed skills to be successful? Success is defined as achieving the desired outcomes.

2. How would you rate the individualization of leader skill development for achieving goals?

For **Resources and Support**, we ask:

1. How well do you assess the emotional and mental well-being of staff?

2. How would you rate utilization of employee assistance resources?

For **Operational Efficiency**, we ask:

1. How effective is [insert Organization Name] at removing barriers that make it easier for people to do their work?

2. How well does [insert Organization Name] identify and implement best practices?

We've completed these assessments with organizations of just about every size, shape, and function within healthcare. Each time we've completed one, leadership teams tell us that it helps make priorities even clearer, in terms of where they should focus immediately versus trying to take on all things related to their retention and engagement efforts.

Here's how the assessment process works:

1. We meet with the senior team so they can first see and become familiar with the ecosystem: its components and its ultimate goal of driving engagement and sense of belonging.

2. We then send the survey to the group of leaders the team identifies (we suggest a larger group versus a smaller one). We find each organization easily identifies the group. Often it is those who attend leadership sessions.

3. Once assessments are complete, we begin to assemble the feedback in two ways:

a. A placemat, or large-format visual that is easy to read and translate regarding the responses and what they indicate. Please scan the QR code or visit https://healthcareplussg.com/resources/books/rewiring-excellence/ to see an example.

   b. A presentation designed to create active conversation among the entire leadership team.

4. As we discuss the results for each set of questions, our guidance is for the leaders to avoid the temptation to focus first on the lower scores and/or outliers. The key element of the visual is the distribution curve…Does it lean left? Does it lean right? Is it closer to a perfect bell curve, and where does the peak of the distribution fall? These answers begin to give a senior team and their middle leaders a sense of where the variance lies within their organization. It also begins to give them a sense of prioritization.

In cases where leaders' responses tend to cluster to the right (higher scores/higher current performance), that element is less likely an immediate priority. For those responses that either show a wide spread of answers or cluster to the left (lower scores, poorer current performance), that element is more likely to emerge as a priority. In almost every case where the assessment has been taken, two or three of the elements of the ecosystem emerge as priorities for focus.

For example: In conducting a recent ecosystem assessment for a large regional health system, we found the results for "Selection and Onboarding" and "Resources and Support" skewed to the left (scoring lower in the leaders' opinion) and thus emerged as two significant priorities. When we allowed the leaders in a training session to pose suggestions for improving both areas, the conversations were healthy and helpful. Interestingly, the responses to the other elements from that system were widespread in terms of distribution, indicating a very low sense of alignment across the system.

In another ecosystem assessment for a system that is considered a high-performing organization, the responses for each element tended to lean to a tight distribution to the right (8s, 9s, and 10s)…except one: Skill Building and Career Development. The CEO commented that it wasn't a surprise and validated the decision they had made to pursue external assistance to take leader development to the next level.

No two organizations are exactly the same. These "rewired assessments" become very healthy conversations. Sometimes there are surprising results. Often, results will serve as validation for senior teams' perspectives of the organization. Without fail, someone from the ranks of the middle leaders will say something like, "It was good to be asked," or, "It was nice to have our input valued."

Throughout the next chapters, we'll go deeper on what we've learned about each component of the Human Capital Ecosystem, and, more importantly, a few tips and tactics for each as you decide where your priorities lie.

If you're interested in conducting this assessment, scan this QR code or visit https://healthcareplussg.com/resources/books/rewiring-excellence/.

## The Human Capital Ecosystem: A Deeper Dive

You'll see from the illustration that each element of the ecosystem is connected to each of the other five as well as the center or "hub," which is ultimately an engaged workforce with a high sense of belonging. As we review the Human Capital Ecosystem, we'll go deeper on some of the elements that call for more rewiring than others. Let's get started.

## ECOSYSTEM ELEMENT 1: Selection and Onboarding

How can we improve the selection process? How can we make sure the new person is successful once they begin in their role? With the staffing challenges our industry faces right now, these are urgent questions. So many new hires leave before their first year is up, and many leave in the first few months. By rewiring parts of our selection and onboarding processes, we can begin to reverse this trend.

It is so important that we ask the right interview questions. We need to discover both what the new hire is looking for in their leader and coworkers (this helps create that all-important sense of belonging that leads to full engagement) and also whether the person truly "fits" in terms of values and expectations.

Also, continuous onboarding is crucial. Aramark Healthcare+ has found that the first stay conversation needs to happen on day one. Outside the industry, Southwest Airlines invests heavily in onboarding. They make many connections with new employees the first year to get them engaged in the culture, and it pays off with extremely low voluntary turnover (under 3 percent). As we discuss in Chapter 3, onboarding can actually start during the interview process.

The idea is to make sure the person, beginning at the first interview, feels "This is the place for me."

## ECOSYSTEM ELEMENT 2: Supervisor Relationship

For years most of our focus has been on the relationship between a supervising leader (typically a director or manager) and their team. We often quoted the phrase, "People don't leave their job; they leave their boss." While this can occasionally be true, recent research conducted by Katherine Meese, PhD, at the University of Alabama at Birmingham suggests that there are other factors at play, especially since early 2020. It's clear from this research that there is a stronger correlation of indication to remain with an organization relative to how teammates feel about senior leadership. Trust is the significant key factor.

So, for this part of the Human Capital Ecosystem assessment, we ask the question, "Are middle leaders getting what they need from senior leaders?" This is important for two reasons: 1. Middle leaders still need everything we've coached around the value of a healthy relationship with a one-up leader. 2. Middle leaders are more likely to be able to position senior leadership teams in a positive light to their teams if they feel that fundamental trust in the executive team based upon those relationships with their one-ups. We've talked about a dynamic called "we/they" for a number of years, and we now know the key factor to eliminating we/they is ensuring that the senior-most leaders are paying attention to the needs of middle leaders:

1. Paying close attention to how well we cascade communication clearly and simply from the senior team

2. Keeping commitments of regular one-on-one meetings and having a consistent agenda that includes learning and development (more about that in a later section)

3. Helping middle leaders answer tough questions that come up from the front line

If you think about the research mentioned above and the concept of we/they, trust emerges as an essential driver of relationships up and down the org chart. A great illustration of the impact of trust building and maintaining was the fact that during the pandemic, some leadership teams made it a point to be physically present and visible throughout the organization. While there were early instructions to maintain physical distance or even isolation, the most creative of senior teams found a way to bridge the distance factor. As we emerged from the pandemic, it became clear that it was those organizations whose employees have given much higher ratings of trust and are less prone to "we/they" symptoms.

## ECOSYSTEM ELEMENT 3: Coworker Relationship

In our work over time, we probably emphasized this element less than some of the others related to leadership. However, the last three years have shown beyond a shadow of a doubt its importance when it comes to creating a sense of belonging in a healthcare organization. It seems that more people get the meaning of the question that Gallup used for years in their employee surveys: "Do I have a best friend at work?"

As the pandemic set in, we found the workforce divided by physical location: remote work and work that could never be done remotely. It seems this became the newest version of "we/they." Some individuals' roles could easily be performed remotely, while clearly the clinical work required physical presence within hospitals, clinics, post-acute facilities, and the like. Another dynamic impacting coworker relationships that emerged was an explosion in the use of temporary staff. This creates its own difficulties at times.

Here's an excellent example of how we might rewire these relationships. What if, a week or so prior to temporary staff's arriving, a questionnaire was distributed to them and the permanent team in the department?

The questions for the permanent staff ask: 1. *What are you looking for in a temporary or agency teammate for the next 13 weeks? 2. What would you like them to know about your team and your department?*

The questions for the temporary staff ask: 1. *What are you looking for in a working environment during your 13-week assignment? What would you like the permanent team to know about you…both personally and professionally?*

The completed questionnaire is provided for both sets of teammates…with the express intent to "pre-build" the relationships. That's rewired!

The second element of coworker relationships in the assessment is focused on relationships between departments. This is one area that many organizations have tried to hardwire over the years. Yet it seems they struggled to maintain the focus, especially as the pandemic set in. So rewiring is perhaps a new view of interdepartmental relationships that are somewhat like open-book tests.

There was a nursing instructor in a nursing school in northeast Oklahoma who was known as both the toughest AND best instructor in the program. Interestingly, she also gave the most frequent number of open-book tests. We all remember showing up for class and finding out it was an open-book test. That was a good day! And yet, we graduate and begin our professional careers and we can forget the value of open-book tests. This is a great opportunity for departments that support other departments to take advantage of the open-book test environment.

Often, we've heard that when these departments hear from the departments they support, it's a crisis management interaction, focused on the fire that needs putting out today. It rarely includes healthy, problem-solving-type conversations. The solution is giving support services leaders and their teams the "answers to the test" so they are very clear on expectations.

So…what if the leaders of the support services departments rounded on the leaders of the departments they serve and had a conversation that sounds like this: *I want to be a 9 or 10 on a 10-point scale when you think of the way we support you. Over the next 90 days, what items would you like me to focus on with my team so that when we have this conversation again, we have earned a 9 or 10?*

This rewired conversation allows for a few things to be put in place between the two leaders: *clarity, priority,* and *focus*. Clarity: It's a first-person conversation, not the second-hand, water-cooler kind of talk that can often occur. Priority: It's not 100 things to be improved…it's three (or less!). This also relates to the "Is it doable?" conversation you've seen throughout this book. Focus: The support services department can narrow their own scope of work in a typically already-busy day, which lightens their loads as well.

A final thought: Forging strong coworker relationships builds the leaders of the next generation. Rewiring these basic dynamics allows leadership teams to watch up-and-comers begin to emerge.

## ECOSYSTEM ELEMENT 4: Skill Building and Career Development

Of all the elements that we have seen the need to rewire, skill building and career development is the most significant. The latest research indicates that employees, particularly Generation Z and Millennials, are more likely to stay in a position when they feel their skill building and career development are prioritized. Yet it's not one-size-fits-all. It's important to take an "N=1" approach, which acknowledges that every person has their own unique needs. Our framework includes very specific techniques to make sure people feel invested in, which leads to better retention. This ecosystem element is another one that is so significant that we're devoting an entire chapter to this topic.

## ECOSYSTEM ELEMENT 5: Resources and Support (Well-Being)

There's been additional stress and trauma in every organization after the past few years. This has led to a renewed focus on mental health/wellness. In healthcare, we're fortunate to offer great benefit packages and a variety of user-friendly mental health and well-being resources. However, even after the enhanced emphasis that so many organizations have placed upon well-being, only a small percentage of individuals use them. By removing the stigma around mental health and training leaders to create safe environments for sensitive conversations, we can ensure people get the help they need. And by mastering the tools and tactics that replenish cultures, we can create the kinds of organizations where mental health issues and burnout are less likely to take hold and people are more likely to utilize the well-being resources available.

The real rewiring that shows up in the assessment is to surface the questions and conversations about utilization. The first question also lends to the ability of the senior team to establish and maintain trust with the entire team. How well *do* we assess the emotional and mental well-being of our staff? Our recent work has focused not so much on a deep set of diagnostics, but rather on easy-to-have conversations that create a safe space for supervisors and teammates to get to the heart of each other's well-being. One of the most popular versions of this conversation is using the battery question you'll read in the chapter on rewiring rounding (see Chapter 4).

The other is to rewire the way we begin meetings. What would happen if, instead of jumping right into the thick of the agenda, we took a few minutes to conduct replenishing conversations? If we have a number of new members on the team—or if the group is a newly formed one—build familiarity with replenishment conversations like "Why did you get into healthcare?" "Why do you stay?" "Why do you stay HERE?" Alternately, what if we asked meeting attendees to share one item for which they are grateful prior to the meeting officially beginning? Well-being is connected to a sense of purpose and gratitude, so the more we can inspire these feelings in employees, the better!

The second question in the assessment has to do with asking leaders across the organization how they rate utilization of employee assistance resources. What we've realized is that there is a great opportunity to provide leaders data on utilization so they can understand what is working and opportunities for improvement (OFIs).

## ECOSYSTEM ELEMENT 6: Operational Efficiency

Great organizations make sure that, to the extent they can, they have the systems, equipment, and staffing to allow people to do their best work. No one is perfect, but are we improving? Are we proactively removing the "pebbles in the shoe" that wear people down over time? Are we communicating our actions so people feel their concerns are listened to—and that we care about giving them a workplace that works?

As you might begin to assess, so many of the other elements of the Human Capital Ecosystem can support or detract from operational efficiency. So the first question we might ask is about removing barriers in a way that makes it easier for people to do their work. The second question is on the opposite end of the pendulum swing of efficiency: capturing the good stuff that happens every day and finding ways to scale it across the entire organization. We call this effort "identifying, harvesting, and scaling the bright spots." In almost every organization with which we work, there's an individual, a department, or even an entire region or division that does something really well…and better than the rest of the organization. The challenge is to not allow these best or better practices to occur in isolation, but to flourish across the organization. As with most of our examples in this chapter, the work begins with a good diagnosis.

## Pulling the Ecosystem Together

Now that you've been "around" the ecosystem, the most important takeaways are:

1. Would an assessment like this serve our team?

2. Can we use this kind of assessment to prioritize our time and energy?

3. Are we ready to let go of things that might be long-time habits/approaches but just aren't producing outcomes and consider rewiring our thoughts and approaches for NOW?

If you and your executive leadership team are interested in conducting this assessment or learning more about the Human Capital Ecosystem, scan this QR code or visit https://healthcareplussg.com/resources/books/rewiring-excellence/.

In a way, this book is a journey through some of the most vital parts of the Human Capital Ecosystem. In the next chapter, we'll delve more deeply into how we can rewire the way we select and onboard talent. Then, we'll move on to discuss some other crucial components of the ecosystem that could potentially be rewired. Thank you for reading so far…now let's move forward.

CHAPTER 3

# Rewiring the Selection and Onboarding Processes

In creating the Human Capital Ecosystem™, Engaged (Belonging) was placed at the center, which all components revolved around. During Selection and Onboarding is when belonging truly begins. While we observed in the previous chapter that each element is connected and can influence each of the others, the staffing challenges that the industry faces (and the potential solutions to solving those challenges) start in the Selection and Onboarding process.

Let's look at the data around selection. Most organizations go to great lengths to get hiring right. They screen applicants and interview those people who seem to be a good fit. The leader they will report to then interviews the applicant. The goal is to be comfortable that the skill set is present, or at least the ability to acquire the needed skills. Then the potential coworkers meet with the applicant. If all goes well, the job offer is made and accepted.

The person is excited about the job, or they would not have taken it. Yet despite the hard work, the highest percentage of departures are people who leave within the first year. Some will exit in the first 90 days. A few won't even come back for day two. Some will accept the job and not show up on day one. This creates the opportunity here to rewire the Selection and Onboarding process.

It's not usually necessary to change the entire hardwired system. Much of it can be left in place.

So, what steps lend themselves to rewiring? Again, narrowing the scope to less is important. You might have all applicants watch a video of staff explaining the values and standards of the organization. The idea is to use examples that help the applicant see early on if they want to go to the next step.

During the leader interview, ask these four questions:

*If you are offered this position and you accept it, as your supervisor what can I do so you enjoy working with me?* In essence, you're asking what they are looking for in you, their leader.

*What are you looking for in your coworkers? What characteristics in those you work with will help you feel good about being on the team and part of the family?*

These two questions have a big impact. They're a way of showing interest in what the person needs from the organization, versus starting out with what they bring to it. That comes next.

*As your supervisor, what can I expect from you?* If the person is unsure of the question, be specific. Cover items like attendance, standards, skills, comfort in sharing concerns and asking questions, and so forth.

*Six months from now, what will your coworkers be telling me about working with you? What type of coworker will you be?*

These questions will quickly let both sides know, "Does this job make sense for this person?" If you feel comfortable, you can share the onboarding process and dig into belonging. "What will need to happen for you to feel, *This is the place for me; I am so glad I took this job?*"

If leaders feel comfortable with the answers to these questions, the peer interviewing process will likely be fine. The key is to see if the applicant connects with the peers. We do like it when the applicant completes a quick assessment tool called Management By Strengths (MBS). It helps the person learn more about themselves. It is also very valuable for the team to know how the person tends to work, by zeroing in on four traits (Directness, Extroversion, Pace, and Structure) and determining four preferences (results- or outcome-oriented, team- or people-oriented, timing- or process-oriented, and detail- or structure-oriented). Staff love the tool, it builds teamwork, and it is not expensive.

## Helping People Want to Stay

We were in an organization that was not a large one, yet they told us that 60 people in the past year had accepted a job yet did not show up on day one. Onboarding can help solve this problem. It starts in the interview process. Research shows people are most likely to stay when they feel they are receiving skill and career development. Make sure a skill development conversation is part of the hiring process. Connect consistently with the person prior to day one, from texting to sending a short video of coworkers expressing how excited they are to have the person join the team. Joi, a leader at TriHealth in Cincinnati, Ohio, sends a text with parking instructions and lets the new hire know what door to enter. She includes a reminder to bring their badge. When they arrive, she is waiting at the door for them.

At orientation, share a video on the normal feelings a new person may experience, from excitement to doubt. We provide a five-minute video on this subject. Scan the QR code or visit https://healthcareplussg.com/resources/books/rewiring-excellence/ to get free access to the video.

Here is another orientation technique to try when co-mingling people brand new to their first healthcare job with those with experience. Often a new nurse grad will be nervous; in fact, if they are not, it is unusual. Even though they have had clinical rotation, the first day as a nurse is different. In the orientation, there will be experienced nurses who are new to the organization. To start the day out, ask the experienced nurse to think about their very first job as a new grad and share how they felt. When they do, the room changes. The experienced nurses end up with heightened empathy for the new grads, and the entire time in orientation shifts. The new grads don't feel so alone. They realize "others felt like this."

## Onboarding: The Next Rewiring Opportunity

It is common for organizations to work hard to make sure a new person learns the job. Often they are assigned a buddy or a preceptor. This is a coworker to assist the person in acclimatizing to the role and the team, a safe person to talk with. It is a mentor-type role. As our good friend Katie Boston-Leary, PhD, says, let's make sure the person

## REWIRING THE SELECTION AND ONBOARDING PROCESSES

is a mentor and not a tormentor. We have found that not everyone is good at teaching. They may be very good at the job themselves; however, teaching may not be their strength. The MBS works well in this situation because the mentor knows the best way the person learns.

It also helps to provide education on how to best support the new person. For example, explain that words like *easy* and *simple* don't work well. What is easy or simple to an experienced person may not be easy or simple to a new hire. It also helps if the mentor shares their own story about being new. The new person can feel, *I will never be this good*, and the mentor can assure them that they will.

Also, set up systems for those in the preceptor role to meet and learn from each other. Connect them back to the great purpose they serve. Through those they teach, hundreds and thousands of people's lives are touched.

In my first book, *Hardwiring Excellence* (now published by Huron), I recommended 30- and 90-day new employee meetings. The questions to ask are, *How do we compare to what you felt the first 30 days would be like? Do we match what we said we would be like? Based on where you have worked before, are there things we could implement here?* (People appreciate being able to give input.) *Is there any reason causing you to question if this is the right job and/or the right place for you?* Other questions are, *How can I be helpful to you? Do you feel you are receiving the training you need to learn the job?* These questions should vary based on the person and situation. However, some have taken these questions to mean, *These are the only questions to ask*, or, *These are the best questions to ask*. That was never the intention. The idea is to fit the questions to what makes sense.[1]

A leader who had read one of my books sent an email. They shared that they and those they work with are tired of the same questions and asked for recommendations. My reply was to change the questions (along with an apology for having written them in a way that made readers feel there were no other options). Adjust the questions to each situation. See what works best. Finally, share what is working with others. We all need to be in on making care better. We are on the same team.

In addition to rewiring the questions, you might need to rewire the timing. Our work with Aramark Healthcare+ is a good example. We're very grateful to spend time with Aramark Healthcare+, the healthcare division of Aramark, which provides food services, environmental services, and patient transport services to hospitals all across the U.S. and around the world. Bart Kaericher, their president and CEO, is the type of person we love working with. Here's a story that illustrates why. Tragically, on July 4, 2022, in Highland Park, Illinois, someone shot people at the parade. Seven people were killed, and 48 were injured. Many of the victims were taken to Highland Park Hospital. Aramark staff members, including environmental services professionals, dealt with this tragedy. Bart got on a plane and immediately went to the hospital. He wanted to be with the staff. He did not bring a public relations person and did not post things on social media on what he had done. He just did it. That is what leadership is. Taking the right action in the right way.

But back to our onboarding story. We met Bart and the senior team. We did lots of rewiring based on a diagnosis. Like many, Aramark Healthcare+ had more staff departures than they would like during the pandemic. (They would like none, by the way, unless it is for a person's career advancement.) So, the decision was made to pilot 30-day stay conversations. It was determined that the results could be shared at an upcoming larger session in a few months. We had the timing and questions ready. So, what happened? An adjustment had to be made. During COVID-19, most hotels shut down. Many of the new hires inside Aramark Healthcare+ hospitals started coming in from hotels. On the first day in the hospital job, they experienced things they were not prepared for. Though it was explained that there would be people in the beds (unlike when they cleaned hotel rooms) and that they would need to take lots of safety precautions, hearing it and experiencing it are two different things. What was learned in the first stay conversation had to be rewired to day one. Then, based on that conversation, the next one may be soon afterward. A person might have experienced five more stay interviews before their 30$^{th}$ day. In other words, an action that worked in the past, like 30- and 90-day meetings, needed to be rewired.

Make a big deal out of milestones, especially during that first year. Learn from other programs that focus deeply on retention, like substance abuse recovery. A person in recovery gets a 24-hour medallion (often called a "chip") on day one. Then, in 30-day increments, they receive different colored chips. Everyone claps, and they feel good. At year one, they get heavy metal: a coin with a "1" on it. The person is then asked to share how they did it. Thereafter, a person gets a coin with the next number to commemorate each year of sobriety. Like staying on a job, if a person stays in recovery for that first year, it greatly improves their chances of staying after that. We can learn so much from others.

Those organizations that can either solve or incrementally improve Selection and Onboarding will be the first to emerge in performance in financial/clinical outcomes/safety. We've always known (and have validated with credible data) that healthcare organizations with lower turnover (especially in the patient-facing areas) avoid the higher cost of temporary staff, but most importantly, they have better clinical and operational outcomes like length of stay and mortality rate. Consistency equals high performance…and the best path to consistency is hiring well and retaining better than we ever have before.

CHAPTER 4

# Rewiring Patient and Employee Rounding

Rounding has been a part of healthcare for a long time. My introduction to it was the practice of a physician rounding on patients. Physicians round to make sure the patient is progressing as expected, to answer questions, to adjust the care plan as needed, and to determine when the patient can leave the hospital. Part of rounding is about checking the patient's vitals and communicating with the patient and family.

At Holy Cross in Chicago, when we began to study leader behavior, we felt the term "rounding" fit. Leaders regularly checked in with staff, physicians, and patients. Once we began to hardwire a leader rounding practice, we started to realize that other adjustments needed to be made. How could the leader have time to round? How could leaders in those areas that do not have direct patient contact round—or did they need to? It was a learning process.

Looking back on that time, it's clear that the fact that leader rounding was new to everyone is what kept it from being too complicated. We even coined the term "one question at a time." We also made sure that there were fewer meetings that managers had to attend, including setting "no meeting" windows. It worked, and it worked well.

As described in Chapter 1, rounding proved beneficial. Then, with good intentions, one question became two. Then it became three, then four, then five, then more questions. Paper rounding logs were added to help with follow-up. Later, the question was, "Can rounding logs be automated?" Today, many leaders have found that the rounding process has grown so much that it has become overwhelming.

If rounding is working for you the way it is, great. My experience is managers can look at the rounding software in the same way that physicians look at the electronic health record. Documentation of patient care when there are multiple touchpoints makes a system of documentation helpful, but leader rounding is not in the same vein. We are finding good success from asking leaders to provide a short summary of what was learned each week versus a complicated documentation system. It is doable.

The main question is, "Is what is being asked of the manager doable?" For example, in the inpatient area, what we are finding doable is rounding on new admits, and, if time permits, those patients who are soon to be discharged. The same is true with documentation. We always want the manager to be the main part of the decision on what is doable, whether we're talking about outpatient areas, emergency departments, or medical offices. The collaborative approach works well everywhere in finding the magic of doable. In working with hundreds of managers, when the above approach is discussed, there is a noticeable sigh of relief, a thank-you-for-listening emotion.

None of this means that adding more questions to the rounding process will not work, or that documentation software is not useful. Again, if it is working for you, keep it. If it is not, consider rewiring. The key is the individual buy-in. When a leader feels listened to and valued, the process works.

It also is effective to say, "Let's pause and see how things go." After the leader feels it is doable, still provide a word of caution: "Once this is implemented, if you find that some parts, or all parts, are not doable, let's discuss what is taking place." The issue could be the leader is dealing with too many new items. It could be timing (i.e., questions like, "Can we wait until after the budget process is done?") or it could be the leader needs help in dealing with some performance issues. The beauty is, it all leads to skill development and thus to better outcomes. And it all leads to leader retention.

## Rewiring What Is Asked During Rounding

I loved the book *Wonder Drug: 7 Scientifically Proven Ways That Serving Others Is the Best Medicine for Yourself*, by Drs. Anthony Mazzarelli and Stephen Trzeciak. It led me to ask, *What is the real question?* The book shared a study by the University of Colorado on the patient's or family member's actual main concern versus what the caregivers perceive as that concern. When researchers asked emergency department patients, "What worries you most?" they received all sorts of answers they didn't expect. In fact, researchers found patients' big worries matched the complaint that brought them into the ED only 26 percent of the time.[1]

This study inspired us to ask, "What is our biggest worry/concern right now?" when rounding on patients and family. It is our number-one recommendation. My belief is that those who work in healthcare are smart and will act on what is heard. Due to my own medical situation, I see my dermatologist team (MD and PA) every month. This is how we start the conversation: "What is your biggest concern? What are you noticing with your skin?" It works.

We also find this approach works well with leaders. Mary Parker Follett (1868-1933) gave birth to the concept of transformational leadership. Her belief, which I agree with, is that trust is the foundation of a great culture. In meeting with leaders, we ask them this: "If you could ask the patients in your area only one question, what would it be?" Generally, there are a wide variety of leaders in the room. One leader might be interested in determining ease of scheduling. Another might be interested in how well pre-survey communication is working. What is so effective is that the leaders feel trusted and respected. This approach creates good conversations, buy-in from leaders, and the understanding that there is flexibility in rounding. The leaders find joy in this method. They also quickly see what is working well and what needs to be changed. They don't feel like they are being asked to communicate like robots.

## Rewiring Employee Rounding

Similar to patient rounding, leader rounding on employees can benefit from rewiring. All rounding is best when it builds relationships. When trust is built, so is a person's willingness to share concerns.

I'm such a huge believer in Relationship Rounding™. This practice, in which you hold regular, one-on-one conversations with employees to see what would make their lives better and see how they're doing mentally and emotionally, gives one the chance to get to know each person as an individual. It helps one find out how they like to work and discover what matters most *to each person*.

Relationship Rounding is meant to build the emotional bank account. It is being interested versus interesting. It is taking time to know what is important to each staff person. It means connecting first on a personal level prior to the task at hand. It creates the feeling, "My boss and my organization care about me as a person."

My suggestion is to put a Relationship Rounding practice in place right away. The sooner you get to know employees as individuals, the better. If someone makes a request, follow up with action *if at all possible*. If you can't meet a request, explain why and ask, "What else could we do that would help?"

One question that works well during Relationship Rounding is the battery charge question. Replace asking the employee, "How are you?" each day with, "If you were a phone, what would your current charge percentage be?" The phone battery question leads to a much deeper conversation. It just hits people in a different way.

Consider how we care for our phones. We buy protective gear for them. We decorate them with everything from sparkles to school colors. We don't let them get too hot or too cold. We may put a tracker on them so they don't get lost. Our phones are often the last thing we see before falling asleep and the first thing we connect with in the morning. We make sure all steps are taken to keep our phone charged. (Want to see separation anxiety? Observe someone in an airport who realizes they don't have a charger!) In short, we tend to take much better care of our phones than we do ourselves.

We learn a lot when we ask people what their battery charge is at any given time. There are some who routinely have a higher charge and others who are a bit lower. Some are more consistent, and some vary. We have been sharing this question in workshops. We regularly get notes from leaders on how this rewire of "How are you?" to the battery question gets such different responses. One department likes the battery process to the point that the staff decided at each shift to have each person write their battery charge on the whiteboard. It builds the sense of team.

Healthcare people are so helpful. If during a huddle, a person says their battery charge is low, the team wants to know how they can help. We also find that more than half the time, the lower battery charge is related to a personal issue, not a work item. It can range from a bad night of sleep from too much caffeine to worrying about a family member. Often, it's a short-term issue that will resolve itself. Other times, it leads to a discussion on what is available to help the person.

Providing recognition is another way to engage people and build strong relationships. Another good question to ask during rounding is how a person likes to be recognized or when they feel the most valued. People are different. Even if a person says they don't like recognition, they may be thinking of public recognition. Many introverts don't enjoy this. However, most people like feeling appreciated. The key is to individualize it to the person's comfort level.

The key in all of this is to take a fresh look at the approaches being used. If what you are doing is creating great employee and physician engagement, and a great patient experience, keep doing what you are doing. If not, it is time to rewire. It does not mean that what was in place at the time was wrong. It does mean times have changed.

I remember when my workplace got its first fax machine. Some of you may not even know what they were. The fax machine was a device in which information came over the wire and was duplicated on paper. We looked at the first fax like we were watching a birth. A miracle. This made sense at the time, yet the fax machine is obsolete today.

The same is true with some of the methods used for improving the patient experience and employee and physician engagement. One of my past company's early clients was Sharp HealthCare. They kicked off the Sharp Experience in the San Diego area 20-plus years ago. The goal, which they achieved, was to make sure patients, employees, and physicians had great experiences. Was it perfect? No, nothing is. Was it much better than previous approaches? Yes. As you can see, even the word "experience" is not new in healthcare. The point is not the word as much as the feeling a person gets.

Let's keep the rewiring conversation going.

> *In order to provide a voice from the field, we asked Lisa Reich, RN, with Healthcare Plus Solutions Group, to provide her perspective on how rounding on patients has evolved over the years, how HCAHPS changed things, and what we can do to make patient perception of care better and better.*
>
> ### Let's Fertilize the Garden, Not Dig in the Dirt. (A Guest Perspective on Rewiring Patient Rounding)
> #### by Lisa Reich, RN
>
> I have watched patient rounding transform. When it started, it was really fun. We'd go into a patient room and talk with them—just relaxed conversation. But then, patient experience increased in importance, and organizations were expected to demonstrate their great care by a score, and the word "score" is not what excites healthcare workers. They are not about scores. They are about helping people. Suddenly, rounding grew legs!
>
> More consistent patient check-ins by me, the manager, helped. If I found problems before the patient left, I could fix

them. We are great "fixers" in healthcare. Our brains seem to be wired to look for what is wrong (the diagnosis) so we can get right to the treatment part. This is good in medicine, but not so good in human relationships.

Pretty soon this "rounding" process had all kinds of things tied to it. I started looking at patient responses and tried to proactively address survey items by dropping key words. This also led to some great intentions and may have even worked for a while! Then I thought we could use electronics to have data available to study and learn from—again, an admirable intent and idea!

Some of us (and yes, I mean me specifically) fumble with technology. I feel a bit awkward when I have to type and talk. My talking becomes a little more like *reading* rather than *discussing*. Suddenly, topics to discuss turned into, "Are we or are we not doing this?"

In our country, hospitals do HCAHPS surveys as a standardized way to measure patients' perspectives of the care they receive. (As you probably know, HCAHPS stands for Hospital Consumer Assessment of Healthcare Providers and Systems, and was developed by CMS and AHRQ beginning in 2002 and implemented in 2006.) Nationally, results have remained relatively flat for about the last six or seven years—with a lot of people working really hard to make it better.[2] So, it seems rewiring is in order.

However, rewiring rounding in light of HCAHPS is a lot easier in thought than in action.

Here is a suggestion: Why don't we start by sharing with the patient all the things we are doing to ensure care is great? Not, "How often was your room and bathroom kept clean?" Possible responses are *always, usually, sometimes,* and *never.* Most organizations get a lot of usually and sometimes responses.

But what would happen if we share with the patient things done to ensure their room is cleaned and sanitized? How about if we go in the bathroom and look at it (we don't need to white glove it)—just so they know one time (at least) during their stay someone cared enough to ensure that the bathroom was clean? And what if we told them it was clean, by saying, "Our environmental service tech cleans and sanitizes each room every day. They sanitize the surfaces like your bedside stand, sink, and counters. They clean the floor and remove the trash. They sanitize the bathroom. I can see your room looks clean and sanitized (as you look around to be sure it was done). How has it been for you while you have been here?"

This is much different from, "Has your room been cleaned?"

Sometimes when I look at the questions hospitals are asking their patients in rounding, I see we are "digging in the dirt." We are still focused on finding something wrong so it can be fixed. Let's start to highlight what we are doing well instead—in other words, let's fertilize the garden we are already tending.

Instead of asking if the nursing team does routine purposeful rounding, let's flip it around and tell them what we do and why, then ask them how it's been—e.g., something like this from the manager: "Our nursing team is committed to meeting your needs by taking care of things you may need while they are in the room. This is why they are [insert what takes place]."

Lay out expectations for responsiveness. "It will usually take about [insert what is the norm for your specific area] minutes to answer a call light. This allows enough time to finish with one patient and properly clean hands to go to the next room. How have we done for you?" This is more concept rounding than scripted rounding. We're really trying to highlight what we do rather than asking *if* we did it or not. We're asking questions in an open format with this concept: *Here is what we do and why. How has that been for you?*

We have truly wonderful people who are doing patient rounding, people who sincerely care about the patient. Each one of them is different, with a wide diversity of personalities and approaches. Let's let those differences shine through! Let them be them! Certainly, giving some ideas for what the rounding might sound like is needed, and helping them practice it will help them rewire this rounding process. Patients will remember how the people they interacted with treated them. This is where the human-to-human part becomes really important.

Look at the number of points (or questions). It is obvious: We cannot hit every topic. These patients are sick and in the hospital! Our rounding should normally take two to three minutes, not five to ten minutes. Work with what our patients have already told us through our HCAHPS survey data and determine where we have previously had deficits in communicating our care. If we really have quality-of-care issues, we need to fix those. Most of the time, we are doing the work already—the patient is just not aware of it.

Before you rewire anything, is what you are doing working? For some of you, yes, it's working just fine. If so, don't change it. But if you aren't satisfied with the outcomes, consider rewiring. Remove some of the obstacles. Maybe start with your rounding template (paper or electronic)—and if you aren't using the data, maybe you just need to use it as a guide to the conversation and a place to write down anything important to follow up with. Maybe you just need to motivate the rounding to happen; if that's the case, keep track of whom you rounded with in the tool.

Rewire. Try this new concept approach on one unit for a month or two. See if it makes a difference! If not, reevaluate. A hard part is to stop doing things that are no longer working well. Just because it worked at one time or worked at another location, does not mean it will work now or on your unit.

Remember to really think about what you are trying to communicate. One of the questions I see often is, "Do you know the name of _____ [insert your nurse, your housekeeper, etc.]?" I am not sure why we started asking that, and honestly our patients aren't sure either…however, if we give our intent behind giving our name to our patients (introducing ourselves), then it has meaning. For example: "You may have noticed that I introduced myself and knocked before I came into your room. At XX Hospital, we feel your room is your space, and we want to be respectful of you. How has that been?" Now you've told them why you knocked and introduced yourself… so now it has meaning. And isn't that really why we do it?

Our teams do great work, each and every day with thousands of patients. Our intent is nearly always pure—to provide excellent care for our patients. Let's highlight that care—I say, let's fertilize the garden instead of digging in the dirt!

# CHAPTER 5

# Rewiring Leader Development

It is exciting to see the impact precision medicine—an approach that tailors treatment to individual differences in patients—is having on improving clinical outcomes. This does not mean past methods were not the best at the time. It does mean that as more is learned, changes are made to improve patient care.

My own experience with being on the receiving end of precision medicine has helped me understand how an individual's makeup will impact the care that is received as well as the outcome. My oncologist shared with me that a personalized treatment we had to convince an insurance company to cover for my care is now common, and is started much earlier in the treatment process. In other words, in the span of just a few years, what was an experimental treatment has become standard. Precision medicine works.

Marcia Horn, JD, of ICAN, a cancer navigation organization, shared with me the power of the N=1 approach. In statistical terms, everyone is an N of 1, or a unique individual. This resonated with me as it relates to rewiring—and in this case, *new wiring*—the way we help each person optimize their own uniqueness to achieve the outcomes they want from their career.

Years ago, while working in my previous career as a teacher of children with special needs, we looked at each child as an individual. Each child had an individualized education program or an IEP. It makes sense to use the same approach in helping people maximize their own individual human potential.

When asked by people what I hope my impact on healthcare has been, my reply is often around leader development. Mark Clement, then CEO at Holy Cross Hospital in Chicago, introduced this subject to me in 1993. He brought in Clay Sherman, author of *Creating the New American Hospital: A Time for Greatness*, to conduct two days of leadership development every 90 days. The impact on me was significant. My realization was that I was not nearly as skilled as I previously thought. These development sessions exposed me to much better ways of doing things. When the group left the session each 90 days, we were more aligned and consistent. The experience was a life changer for me and certainly for many others. It made me more teachable and hungrier to learn more. Clay Sherman changed my career. Mark Clement, in providing the learning, changed my life.

In the healthcare field, the majority of those who take on their first supervisory role may do so with very little (or no) leadership development beyond experiencing how the person they reported to led. My observation is less than 10 percent of those in a department leadership position have a degree in healthcare administration, an MBA, or a related master's degree. Most of their degrees and/or experience are in the specific area they are working in. It is great that they have experience in the area they are leading, and they do have credibility. They know what it is like to do the job. The big difference is they now have a new job that requires skills they may not have.

Learning those skills takes time. Leaders need to be proficient in hiring (and at times firing), onboarding, development, financial stewardship, service, process improvement, difficult conversations, change management…and the list goes on. We can see a correlation with physicians. Most residencies are three years long, and this is *after* medical school. If it is felt it takes three years for physicians, how long will it take a person new to leadership to feel fully competent? Personally, my journey to be better is still underway.

From 2020 to 2023, the pandemic impacted the ability of organizations to provide leadership skill development in general. Many leaders were in staffing or other pandemic functions. Outside help was canceled or greatly limited due to the inability to gather in person. For many leaders, just the opportunity to learn from peers was not as available due to the limitations the pandemic created. From my own experience as a first-time supervisor, it was so helpful to lean on peers with more experience to ask how to budget, how to handle an employee with an attitude that is not good, and so forth. Often, my classroom was coffee with more experienced peers.

Our early calls at Healthcare Plus Solutions Group were to help recapture what once was, or, as we wrote about in a previous chapter, to get back to basics. While meeting with hundreds of people in leadership, here is what was heard. *We are overwhelmed right now. Yes, we want to improve our skills; however, I am just trying to get my head above water. I feel like I am failing. I don't want people to know how I am struggling. I don't know if I can do this. I already have a full plate.*

From these responses, it is apparent that, for most organizations, development needed to be adjusted. This is why we created the

Precision Leader Development™ (PLD) method, which allows for customized development of the individual.

To clarify, we're not saying development needs to be completely changed. People still get value from the leadership group getting together. Understanding organizational goals is a must in alignment and connecting to purpose. People enjoy the recognition and sharing of success. Getting organizational plans and next steps helps a leader, as well as ways to ensure that the information is cascaded. There are benefits to a general presentation on relevant topics.

As before, leaders are asked to take this information to the organization's various departments and units. The biggest adjustment is the realization that what was previously called development is (and always has been) about education and awareness. Group sessions are good. Today individual or precision development is a difference maker.

The key to rewiring is taking skill building to the individual leader level. As with precision medicine, it is an N=1 strategy. This requires asking, *What skills does the leader need to have for the role they are in at this time? Is the leader aware of their current skill level?* This is where the collaborative approach works. The following figure shows an example of skills, self-rating and supervisor feedback. It's important to realize that the skill that's rated the lowest may not be the highest priority. For example, if a department is small and has little employee turnover, selection skills are not needed at the time.

# HEALTHCARE PLUS SOLUTIONS GROUP

## Leader Skills Rating

This survey is designed to rate your own skill level among the list below.
After you rate yourself, have your direct supervisor rate your current skill level.

Employee name:

Supervisor name:

**FOR CURRENT SKILL LEVEL:**
1 = Opportunity, not skilled, almost no knowledge about the subject
10 = Strength, highly skilled, could teach the subject

### 1. Selection of talent and onboarding
SELF  1 ○  2 ○  3 ○  4 ○  5 ○  6 ○  7 ○  8 ○  9 ○  10 ○
DIRECT SUPERVISOR  1 ○  2 ○  3 ○  4 ○  5 ○  6 ○  7 ○  8 ○  9 ○  10 ○

### 2. Running an effective meeting
SELF  1 ○  2 ○  3 ○  4 ○  5 ○  6 ○  7 ○  8 ○  9 ○  10 ○
DIRECT SUPERVISOR  1 ○  2 ○  3 ○  4 ○  5 ○  6 ○  7 ○  8 ○  9 ○  10 ○

### 3. Understanding financial statements, manage and reduce expenses
SELF  1 ○  2 ○  3 ○  4 ○  5 ○  6 ○  7 ○  8 ○  9 ○  10 ○
DIRECT SUPERVISOR  1 ○  2 ○  3 ○  4 ○  5 ○  6 ○  7 ○  8 ○  9 ○  10 ○

### 4. Process improvement
SELF  1 ○  2 ○  3 ○  4 ○  5 ○  6 ○  7 ○  8 ○  9 ○  10 ○
DIRECT SUPERVISOR  1 ○  2 ○  3 ○  4 ○  5 ○  6 ○  7 ○  8 ○  9 ○  10 ○

### 5. Understanding measurement (employees, customers)
SELF  1 ○  2 ○  3 ○  4 ○  5 ○  6 ○  7 ○  8 ○  9 ○  10 ○
DIRECT SUPERVISOR  1 ○  2 ○  3 ○  4 ○  5 ○  6 ○  7 ○  8 ○  9 ○  10 ○

### 6. Difficult conversations (employees, customers)
SELF  1 ○  2 ○  3 ○  4 ○  5 ○  6 ○  7 ○  8 ○  9 ○  10 ○
DIRECT SUPERVISOR  1 ○  2 ○  3 ○  4 ○  5 ○  6 ○  7 ○  8 ○  9 ○  10 ○

### 7. Talent development
SELF  1 ○  2 ○  3 ○  4 ○  5 ○  6 ○  7 ○  8 ○  9 ○  10 ○
DIRECT SUPERVISOR  1 ○  2 ○  3 ○  4 ○  5 ○  6 ○  7 ○  8 ○  9 ○  10 ○

### 8. Connecting the external environment to internal actions
SELF  1 ○  2 ○  3 ○  4 ○  5 ○  6 ○  7 ○  8 ○  9 ○  10 ○
DIRECT SUPERVISOR  1 ○  2 ○  3 ○  4 ○  5 ○  6 ○  7 ○  8 ○  9 ○  10 ○

### 9. Change management
SELF  1 ○  2 ○  3 ○  4 ○  5 ○  6 ○  7 ○  8 ○  9 ○  10 ○
DIRECT SUPERVISOR  1 ○  2 ○  3 ○  4 ○  5 ○  6 ○  7 ○  8 ○  9 ○  10 ○

### 10. Reward and recognition
SELF  1 ○  2 ○  3 ○  4 ○  5 ○  6 ○  7 ○  8 ○  9 ○  10 ○
DIRECT SUPERVISOR  1 ○  2 ○  3 ○  4 ○  5 ○  6 ○  7 ○  8 ○  9 ○  10 ○

www.HealthcarePlusSG.com

Copyright © 2023 by Healthcare Plus Solutions Group. All rights reserved.

Scan the QR code below or visit https://healthcareplussg.com/resources/books/rewiring-excellence/ to see the figure in more detail and download the template.

Another component in PLD is examining the traits of the individual. Is the person more people-oriented, pace-oriented, or structure-oriented? What is their degree of outcome orientation? What blind spots might they have?

How does the individual learn best? Some people learn better by reading, some by listening. Some are better with one-on-one coaching, while others do well in small or larger group settings. Some learn by doing.

Interestingly, we have learned that what is meant to be helpful can miss the mark. Too much development too soon can be a demotivator, in that the person needs time to practice each skill before moving on to the next.

Then there are other aspects of PLD, such as assessments in critical thinking, the person's ability to process information, and so forth.

The above description may make the process sound more complicated than it is. The goal is to help the person and their leader decide on the desired outcomes, what skills to focus on, and the best approach in development.

To help with this, we created a tool called OSAR™. The O stands for the **O**utcome the person needs to achieve; S is for the **S**kill(s) needed to achieve the outcome; A is for the **A**ctions or steps to be taken to acquire the skill; and R stands for the **R**esources needed for the development. We find this approach is well received by the leader. It makes their skill building doable.

Here is an example of an OSAR Template:

| OSAR™ - EXAMPLE USE |||||
|---|---|---|---|
| **Name:** ||| **Date:** |
| **OUTCOME** | **SKILL(S)** | **ACTIONS** | **RESOURCES** |
| What is the outcome you want to achieve? | What skill(s) do you want to master? | What actions will you take to achieve this outcome? | What resources will be used to build these skills? |
| Reduce 90-day turnover from 31% to 20%. | Selection and early onboarding. | Adjust selection to new, more relevant questions. | New selection questions:<br>- What are you looking for in your supervisor and coworkers?<br>- What can your coworkers and I count on from you? |
| | | Start onboarding process the minute the job is accepted. | |
| | | Get to know the new employee better by discovering their interests, family background, and how they like to spend their free time. This helps you learn their keys to feeling, *This is the place for me.* | Read *The Calling* and connect to each person's sense of place. |
| | | Conduct weekly stay conversations. | Read article about stay interviews. |
| | | Celebrate employee's first 30, 60, and 90 days. | |

Scan the QR code below or visit https://healthcareplussg.com/resources/books/rewiring-excellence/ to see the graphic in more detail.

We suggest the term "investing" in skill building or development be used. It is an investment—one that is desired and one that is likely to pay off in a big way as we seek to build cultures that attract and retain the best talent and lead to the best possible clinical outcomes.

We recently conducted the Models of Care Insight Study in collaboration with the American Nurses Association (ANA) and Joslin Insight. Its purpose was to explore new and alternative models of care to implement across the U.S.

One of the findings was that 92 percent of nurses in leadership positions desire skill development, yet a far smaller percentage feel they are receiving adequate skill development.

Precision Leader Development provides elements of rewiring as well as new wiring on how people receive development. Much like precision medicine is improving the quality of life for patients, PLD improves the quality of life for those working in healthcare.

As Mark Clement, currently the president and CEO of TriHealth, said, "It is a game changer."

# CHAPTER 6

# Rewiring Skill Building and the Evaluation Process

There is overwhelming evidence that all employee retention increases with skill and career development. So does organizational performance. Typically, when leaders are asked, "Do you provide skill and career development to staff?" the answer is "yes." When staff members are asked, "Do you receive skill and career development?" the most frequent answer is either "no" or "not to the level I would like." Not wrong, just different perceptions.

Disconnects like this suggest that the traditional approach to employee development, and the evaluations that measure its success, may benefit from a rewire.

If you've read everything up until now, you might notice we've already broached the subject of skill building. Earlier in the book, we addressed onboarding. In the previous chapter, we covered leader development. Both share rewiring techniques that fall under the category of skill building. In this chapter, we will talk about a few other areas that can use rewiring.

First, a mindset shift may be needed. Who oversees an employee's skill and career development? One quick answer might be "the person themselves." Yes, this is true, to a point. However, most people, including those new in leadership, will not be comfortable asking for the resources for development. Some may point to areas such as human resources, organizational development, or education. These areas do offer valuable resources and support employee development. However, the key developer of an employee is their immediate supervisor. Everyone who leads people is "chief development officer" for those they lead. Some leaders are natural developers of people. They are often described as mentors. Others may find the role doesn't come as easily. It's okay. We can all learn.

As mentioned already, every good organization is always in the process of change or at times reinventing itself. This means looking for ways to improve results. Because something worked in the past does *not* mean it is still working or getting the needed results. At times this is due to external environment changes. There may not be enough time or enough staff or enough money. What's interesting is that the most creative solutions often come from times of disruption. We may continue on with behavior that used to work but no longer does, or that works once in a while, until we have no choice but to change.

This story helped me. A bird was provided food when it hit a button with its beak. The bird quickly learned that every time it hit the button, food came out. Then, in one instance, a change was made: When the button was hit, no food came out. After a while, the bird figured out an alternative way to get food. Why? Because the old way did not work. In another situation, the process was changed. Every once in a while, when the button was hit, food came out. Most of the time, though, it did not. The amount of food dispensed was not enough to be sustainable for the bird. Even so, the bird kept hitting the button more often and did not look for alternative solutions.

Why? Because the button still worked once in a while. This is the same impulse that keeps people and organizations from moving to better ways. There is a reluctance to leave current methods even when they work only part of the time.

My view on the performance evaluation process has evolved. Yes, in my mind, there is still great value in clarity of outcomes. There is great value in knowing priorities. Items like dashboards are important. Yes, trust and verification are important. Rather than the once-a-year deep dive into performance, we suggest moving to more frequent conversations on skill and career development.

Over the years, we have found more frequent development conversations are helpful. At first, this was a change that leaders struggled with. They drifted to more of a performance evaluation conversation versus a development one. My experience is that what you call a conversation, a document, a meeting, or anything else shapes the way it is seen and drives the outcome. Be sure the language used reflects your intent. These are skill-building conversations. Some use the term "retention" conversations. Pick the term that works best for you.

Also, pick the frequency that works for you. If you can do them more often, please do. There are many benefits to holding regular development conversations with employees. For example, it helps keep them engaged. It enables you to catch issues quickly so you can help them course correct. It helps you get to know them better and builds strong relationships. It also makes you more likely to identify bright spots you can celebrate. And these are just a few examples of the benefits of frequent, meaningful conversations.

## A Few Sample Questions to Choose from in Development Conversations

There are no hard-and-fast rules around the questions to ask employees. Here are a few suggestions. Don't ask them all at once; it's better to stair-step them throughout the year. This is a menu to select from.

How do you feel you help the organization carry out our mission and strive to reach our goals?

Looking over your work since the beginning of this year, what have you done well? What are your greatest accomplishments?

Do you feel appreciated?

What are some areas of opportunity you want to improve within your current role? In what area or skill do you feel weak?

Do you feel that your goals/priorities for the rest of the year are clear? How do you feel I can help you achieve them?

What training, education, or activities do you feel would be beneficial to you in your role?

Do you have access to all the tools and/or resources you need to do your job? Is there anything that prevents you from doing the best job you can?

As your leader, what do you feel I do well that is helpful to you? What suggestions do you have to help me be more effective for you?

> How do you like to receive feedback? How do you like to be recognized?
>
> How would you rate your overall satisfaction on a 1-10 scale? How would you rate your engagement?
>
> What can I improve upon?
>
> Do you have any questions for me?
>
> Finally, be sure to remind them of the employee assistance program (EAP) they can use if needed. It's important to have these conversations with all employees.

As mentioned in the previous chapter, we like the word "invest" in connection with offering skill building: "You are being invested in because you are important." Organizations share how important it is to invest regularly in preventive maintenance for equipment, so why not have the same connection to investing in people? We know if we don't regularly invest in our facilities, we will pay a steep price. In creating bond ratings, a rating agency factors in the age of the plant. What if they used something similar for an organization's investment in people?

When presenting at organizations, we will at some point share that this session or day is a retention strategy. The message is: "Your CEO is investing in you." Why? So you feel better about your skill, your role, and the organization itself. Light bulbs turn on in the room. Many did not see the development connection to retention. You begin to see development as an opportunity rather than an obligation. This applies to all skill building. It is a tactic. The goal is great operational results—which we know are dependent on invested-in, retained, engaged, healthy teams.

My book *Sundays with Quint* offers many chapters that help leaders connect the dots for people on the *why* behind what is being done or what you're asking them to do. One can't assume a person sees a development conversation as a good thing if they aren't told why it is happening. This is why leaders need to stay focused on the message, "Development is an investment in your skill and career development, because you are important." Try using the words "skill building" versus "education program." Use "individual development" more often than "organization development."

The way we frame something determines how well people accept and buy into it. Often when outside expertise is brought in for good reasons, some will take it as, "We are not doing a good job." Yes, results may need to be improved. Yet the outside resource is an investment in skill development and needs to be presented that way. Soak up all the help you can.

This approach will help people come to see development as an opportunity, not an obligation. They will be more likely to proactively seek out skill development rather than waiting for you to provide it. They will begin to "own" their development. All of this creates a culture of continuous learning and collaboration that will move your company forward.

As written earlier, clarity of goals is important. By adding continuous skill building and monthly check-ins, these outcomes have a much better chance of being achieved.

Here are a few tips and takeaways to keep in mind:

**Leaders are the overseers of development for those they lead.** Other areas can be good resources; however, the key to development is an employee's leader. Leaders often benefit from skill development on how to best help people achieve their goals. Each leader, when asked, should be able to share, by employee, what skill development is being focused on.

**Feedback is not a once-a-year or twice-a-year event.** Yes, some individuals will naturally pick up skills on their own. Most will appreciate the investment being made in their skills.

**Make development individual.** Group training and predetermined content and hours are important, but bring skill development to the individual level. N=1. Each person is different.

**Shift language to get people focused on the future.** "Continuous quality improvement" is a recognized term. It is not about judging past performance; it's about always looking for ways to get better. Move to "continuous skill development." Also use the word "investing." Like an organization invests in upkeep of a plant and equipment, most also invest in making the workforce better and better. Help people connect the dots.

**Evaluate the resources.** Most organizations are loaded with books, videos, and other skill-building resources. Put a feedback loop in place that provides users the opportunity to rate the value of each resource. It will lead to better consistency.

My take is, the great majority of people bring the will to do well on a job. What they may not have is the skill. By prioritizing skill development, and holding regular conversations around it, we can help them become the high-performing employees they already want to be.

# CHAPTER 7

# Rewiring Physician Ownership

During a workshop, the chief medical officer of a 450 physician and advanced practice provider group was sharing some information. The group was made up of people of diverse ages. One data point that was shared was the percentage of patients who could have received care from someone in the group (medical staff), yet were referred elsewhere for care. The leader then displayed out-migration statistics. Some call this leakage. What it means is that care that could be provided by someone in the group or within the entire medical staff and/or within the system is referred elsewhere. It is a loss of a patient and also a loss of dollars—dollars needed to support patient care, from staff to equipment to facilities.

In preparation for the session, a survey was sent out to the entire group to learn how knowledgeable the individuals were about their peer medical staff members. Some are employed by the system. Some are not employed by the system but are connected via their being on the medical staff. They all benefit if the system does well.

The survey covered items like training, certifications, clinical outcomes, access, etc. The answers to the survey questions ranged from 1-5, with 1 being "unaware" to 5 being "very aware." About 75 percent of the group rated survey items a 4 or 5. It may be just a coincidence, but 25 percent of patients who could have received care in the system were being referred elsewhere. So out of 450 physicians, over 100 were not as aware of the skills of other physicians on the medical staff as well as resources available as the CMO hoped they would be. It's very normal to see these results in today's environment.

As a sidenote, a CEO of another health system contacted me after a medical staff retreat. She was excited about the time the group spent together. She commented on how great it was for many of the physicians to meet for the first time (in person) the physicians they often refer patients to. How things have changed! The familiarity with other physicians surely impacts referral patterns.

Back to the workshop: As the group worked at tables, the conversation was around, "How can we create a sense of ownership when many physicians from a legal standpoint are not owners?"

Not that long ago, most physicians *were* owners, to some extent. They were shareholders in a small professional corporation (PC). In addition, most spent some time at the hospital rounding on patients. This led to their spending time in the physician lounge, in the medical library, and in the physician dining room. This time at the hospital gave physicians the opportunity to become familiar with each other and develop a sense of camaraderie.

Also, due to not having an electronic health record (EHR) to fill out or the use of technology to communicate, people spoke more to each other. Physicians spent lots of time getting to know potential referral physicians prior to EHRs. Like most advances, there can be a negative consequence to some degree.

With regard to hiring, all the physicians in the small group, or at minimum in that area of medicine, were part of the process. At times, the last physician in had veto power over when the next physician would be hired. In a multi-specialty group, a primary care physician was part of the selection of a specialist. A get-together would be held to welcome new members. Because the group took a financial hit until the new physician was busy enough to cover their salary, people were very "bought in" to helping the new addition grow their practice. There were, of course, very large groups that might not be able to do all of the above; however, they still felt a sense of input.

### Dr. Ernie Deeds: A Forerunner to Modern Hospitalists

Ernie Deeds was an internist in Janesville, Wisconsin. He was part of the River View Clinic, a multi-specialty group. The group decided in the 1980s to open a small clinic about 30 minutes from Janesville in Delavan, Wisconsin. The clinic saw patients from that area and wanted to have an eastern presence. Dr. Deeds offered to go to Delavan, on the condition that other physicians would take care of his patients when they were in Mercy Hospital. It made sense. This way Dr. Deeds could also see more patients versus spending time in the hospital. While not called a hospitalist per se—for that term did not come about till the mid-1990s—Dr. Deeds was a forerunner.

I remember the anxiety of the patients as partners of Dr. Deeds oversaw them while in the hospital. Those physicians had to make sure the patient knew they were in touch with Dr. Deeds, for the patient would most likely be discharged back to him. They did this in various ways, from offering verbal

> assurance to writing Dr. Deeds' name on the whiteboard next to their name so the patient knew the physicians were communicating. Also, because Dr. Deeds had been part of the group for years, he knew all the physicians very well. The term "hospitalist" was coined in a 1996 *New England Journal of Medicine* article by Drs. Robert Wachter and Lee Goldman. Dr. Wachter is considered the father of the field by many—but Dr. Deeds should get an assist.

Today most of what is described above is no longer in existence, and the parts that do exist are different. Physicians are very smart, so the fact that things have changed means they understand the shifting sands. Due to insurance contracting, the expense of acquiring and maintaining technology, the expense of maintaining a viable practice, various on-call challenges, and all sorts of other reasons, physician employment situations have changed. Many are part of larger organizations. A physician can be an employee of a health system, a very large medical group, an insurance company, and/or a private equity investor.

There can be many advantages to this shift. It provides access to needed technology. The physician has no personal debt as an owner of a PC. Often they have a better on-call situation, a strong referral network, and so forth. While at times nostalgia creeps in for the good ole days, those days also had issues. The question is this: How can today's environment be rewired so that some of the advantages of the old days are retained along with the new advantages?

One key is not assuming that physicians will naturally refer patients to others in the group simply because they are part of the same organization. Physicians put their patients first. They are not going to refer a patient to another person, department, or so forth unless they feel it is best for the patient. They are not going to change from a known caregiver to an unknown caregiver. Healthcare systems also want patients to receive the very best care.

If you are a physician who depends on referrals, ask yourself, *If I were in private practice, what would I be doing to build a relationship with other physicians?* The days of physicians seeing each other at the hospital, in the physician lounge, the medical library, the in-person clinical medical education session, or the quarterly medical staff function are long gone (or greatly reduced).

Don't assume that referrals and patients will be kept in the network. Even if there are significant financial reasons for staying in network, physicians will refer to whomever they feel will be most helpful to the patient. Monitor patients referred out of network. Why? To learn. Why was the patient referred out of network? Is there an access challenge? Is there an unfamiliarity? Is there a clinical reason? You can then make changes based on what you learn.

At one time, it was not unusual for organizations to employ people to visit members of the medical staff to build relationships and, most of all, make sure the physicians were aware of new members of the medical staff, new technology, and other changes. This was particularly important if members of the medical staff were splitters as well as serving on multiple medical staffs. While these situations are not as prevalent, what was done by medical staff relations personnel is as important now as before.

Organizations also benefit from involving physicians in the hiring process. While with large groups not all physicians will be able to directly participate, there are ways to help them be more comfortable with new hires. For example, provide all physicians with a description of the positions you are looking to fill. Ask for any names they want to recommend. Publicize which physicians will be part of the selection process.

Don't assume new physicians are aware of how to build their practice. We know how valuable patient navigators are. Provide each new physician with a "develop a practice" navigator. This person can help them learn who to connect with, how things work, and how to navigate the twists and turns of building a practice with a heavy emphasis on appreciation. This includes staff relationship building.

A person does not have to be a literal owner to feel a sense of ownership. Most of us know someone who acts like an owner where they work. They are fiercely loyal to the product and the people. They treat resources like their own and are grateful to be part of the organization. There are some who even tattoo the company logo on themselves. Such cultures tend to have the following things in common:

Owners see the numbers, including all financial numbers. Be transparent with data.

Owners have influence over hiring. Be as inclusive as possible in hiring.

Owners are very engaged in the product and the brand. Again, include as many stakeholders as possible in product and brand decisions.

Owners know the truth about what is going well and what is not. It is okay to share items like the percentage of patients who are referred out of network and why.

Successful owners put value first. In the research that became the book *Built to Last*, Jim Collins reported that in studying organizations that had long-term success, all had periods of ups and downs. All faced times when a choice had to be made between values and revenue. Those that chose values, even though it meant a revenue hit, did better in the long run. Those that chose revenue over values did not survive long-term. Putting values first may mean letting a bully go, even though they are a big revenue producer. It may mean making a change that will make people comfortable referring to a physician in the network. It will mean giving up some control over selection and creating numerous ways for people to get to know each other.

Why is it so important to create a sense of physician ownership? For the reason that we are all in healthcare: the betterment of the patient. When physicians are fully engaged and invested, organizations are more successful, cultures are healthier, relationships are stronger, and patients receive better care.

CHAPTER 8

# Rewiring Well-Being

The pandemic brought about a needed increased focus on self-care. Very few people will argue with the statement that those in healthcare take better care of others than they do themselves. Yes, we have all heard the airplane analogy about putting on your own oxygen mask before helping others. Still, it's easy for me to visualize healthcare people continuing to put others' oxygen masks on first! While it makes sense to take care of ourselves first so we have the inner resources we need to be helpful, putting others first is baked into a healthcare worker's DNA.

There is also the stigma around asking for help. While there are good intentions behind the use of words like "resilience" and "heroes," they can also be misinterpreted. The use of *resilience* was never meant to send the message, "Keep going no matter what." Self-care is an important part of being resilient. The same is true with "hero." Yes, there are so many examples of heroic actions by those in healthcare. Yet, again, the word could possibly encourage people to think they have to make a superhuman effort to keep going no matter what. While not up on all the superhero movies, my hope is that they show these superheroes availing themselves of mental health therapy!

Individuals in healthcare are fortunate to work in organizations that offer an array of great resources, from occupational health to wellness and assistance services. The challenge is not lack of resources, which is the case for much of the population. The challenge is to help people feel safe using the resources. My first job in healthcare was in behavioral medicine. I am highly active in the recovery community. A therapist shared with me that I have referred over 100 people to her. Most of these are not from healthcare. People ask why I am so open in sharing my story of alcoholism and recovery. My hope is it helps others overcome the stigma and make use of the resources available to them.

During talks, those in healthcare often share the great resources that they have made available. I was on a panel with chief wellness officers. At the end of the panel, I complimented them on the exceptional array of services available and their passion to make a difference, and then asked about utilization of the services. Each panelist was incredibly open in saying, "That is the biggest issue: the lack of people accessing the well-being services that are available." This is not to say progress is not being made. It is. Can we do better?

Like most in healthcare, my own learning on well-being has increased during the pandemic and a bit before. I wrote a foreword for the book *Why Cope When You Can Heal? How Healthcare Heroes of COVID-19 Can Recover from PTSD*, by Mark Goulston, MD, and Diana Hendel, PharmD. They also wrote another book—*Trauma to Triumph: A Roadmap for Leading Through Disruption (and Thriving on the Other Side)*—that focuses on organizational trauma.

While reading the manuscript to write the foreword for *Why Cope When You Can Heal?*, I recognized my lack of knowledge of trauma. This learning made an impact. Step one is to learn more. Questions began to come up: *What is individual stress? Organizational stress?*

*Individual trauma? Organizational trauma? Can we measure well-being, stress, and trauma in an organization? What is the utilization of resources for those experiencing stress and trauma?* For some of my questions, there were answers. For some, there were not. With that, we went about learning and creating some tools to fill in the gaps.

One solution was to create a 27-minute video to help those in healthcare better understand their well-being, stress, and trauma. You can view this video on the Healthcare Plus Solutions Group (HPSG) website at https://healthcareplussg.com/learning-library/.

Then, to connect this understanding to something everyone is familiar with in healthcare, we created the 1-10 pain scale. People in healthcare are very familiar with the pain scale. We can use the same principle to gauge their emotional temperature. We encourage leaders to use a simple graphic to get a feel for where a caregiver, physician, or staff member is on the spectrum from "Sense of Well-Being" to "Stress" to "Trauma." Ask the person, "If you were evaluating your emotional well-being on a scale from 1 being 'I feel great' to 10 being 'I am not sure I can take it,' what is your pain at this time?"

## TAKING THE TEMPERATURE WITHIN THE ORGANIZATION

- Pain scale as a simple approach

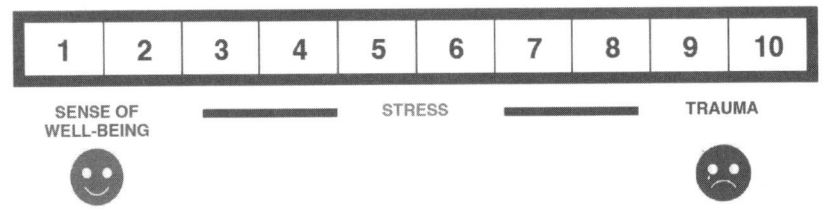

| 1 | 2 | 3 | 4 | 5 | 6 | 7 | 8 | 9 | 10 |
|---|---|---|---|---|---|---|---|---|----|

SENSE OF WELL-BEING — STRESS — TRAUMA

- This gives people a good idea of where the organization is.
- It gives people in the organization an idea that their well-being is on the to-do list.

© Quint Studer

These conversations happen anonymously. It is helpful to break down by work area and role. I was talking to a CEO who did this, and he is so knowledgeable about each area. He shared that one department was a 7.1, which is moving into the early trauma range, while another was in the low 3s, which means people mostly have a sense of well-being with periodic times of stress.

But how do we move to the individual? The Cy-Fair Fire Department in Northwest Harris County, Texas, helped here. They introduced us to a tool from the National Fallen Firefighters Foundation that identifies specific symptoms individuals may be experiencing and helps them pinpoint whether they need assistance. We adapted it with the help of Katherine Meese, PhD, and it will be included in the upcoming book she and I coauthored titled *The Human Margin: Building the Foundations of Trust*.[1]

## Creating Safe Environments for Conversations

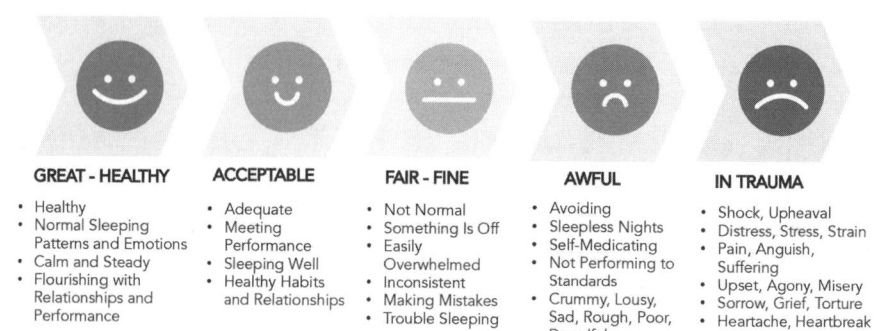

| GREAT - HEALTHY | ACCEPTABLE | FAIR - FINE | AWFUL | IN TRAUMA |
|---|---|---|---|---|
| • Healthy<br>• Normal Sleeping Patterns and Emotions<br>• Calm and Steady<br>• Flourishing with Relationships and Performance | • Adequate<br>• Meeting Performance<br>• Sleeping Well<br>• Healthy Habits and Relationships | • Not Normal<br>• Something Is Off<br>• Easily Overwhelmed<br>• Inconsistent<br>• Making Mistakes<br>• Trouble Sleeping | • Avoiding<br>• Sleepless Nights<br>• Self-Medicating<br>• Not Performing to Standards<br>• Crummy, Lousy, Sad, Rough, Poor, Dreadful, Exhausted | • Shock, Upheaval<br>• Distress, Stress, Strain<br>• Pain, Anguish, Suffering<br>• Upset, Agony, Misery<br>• Sorrow, Grief, Torture<br>• Heartache, Heartbreak |

Adapted from: Stress First Aid for Firefighters and Emergency Services Personnel. National Fallen Firefighters Foundation.

This tool is meant for use in discussing with a person where they are on a well-being to trauma scale. Please do not interpret this as saying everyone in supervision must diagnose each employee's mental state. The opposite is true. Leaders do not diagnose. There are professionals for that. However, they do help the person take a step to see what is causing the pain.

All of these tools are meant to help each person in leadership recognize warning signs as well as create safe conversations with those they work with. A person might watch my video (or read or view whatever educational tools the organization chooses on well-being) and use the 1-10 pain scale. Then they meet with their direct supervisor. They discuss the learnings and review the National Fallen Firefighters Foundation tool. Currently a well-being tool kit is shared and people are given access to a short digital booklet on well-being. You can find all of these resources for free on the HPSG website at https://healthcareplussg.com/learning-library/.

There are times, of course, when the person will share something of a nature that causes the supervisor to be more direct on helping the person access needed professional assistance. Again, the leader is not diagnosing, but serving as a conduit to the right resource.

Depending on your organization, this may be some rewiring to look at. If utilization of helpful resources is low, it may be worth implementing the above. In this case, it is often more of a "new wiring" action than a rewiring one (though it may involve some rewiring). If workforce well-being efforts achieve what you all want, which is healthy people, then they may include minimally hardwiring some of the above recommendations or more.

One more item of note: In this work, we also conducted an anonymous study with physicians. The study showed a high degree of stress and at times trauma combined with an even greater reluctance than other healthcare professionals to seek help.

We would be remiss not to mention the importance of getting to know employees as individuals and creating cultures of engagement and belonging. No two people are alike. The more we know them, the more of a connection we can form—and the stronger that connection, the more likely they will be to tell us the truth about mental health issues.

Of course we know people are more likely to stay when they feel they belong. But also, studies show feeling, *This is the place for me* has positive effects on overall well-being. This is why it is crucial for leaders to regularly ask people: "When do you feel you belong on the unit? In the organization? When do you feel this is the place for you—and are there times when you question that?"

I'd like to close this chapter with a letter I received from Diane McClurg, who recently returned to a job she had retired from in April of 2021. She wrote it after making some changes we suggested, like pitching in to help staff, implementing a morning huddle, recognizing employees, sending thank-you notes, and so forth. She shared that making all these changes had resulted in a greater sense of trust between staff members and in leaders. I feel this letter showcases how the culture change created a sense of belonging that positively impacted everyone's mental health, including her own.

---

Dear Quint,

My last day as interim lab director is August 9. I sincerely want to thank you for sending me *The Well-Being Handbook* and *The Calling*.

I used those two books as my go-to when I thought I was not making progress to get the lab staff to re-engage in how important their jobs are in the care of the patients. When a staff member came and told me she could not "work like this anymore," I shared that I felt that way when I walked back into the lab after having retired from a 40-year career here.

She then shared that she had no clue that I was feeling depressed and upset and wanted to know what I did. I told her that when I put on that lab coat, walked out into the lab, and started processing patient samples, that I reminded myself that I was again part of a team that does really good work. I told her I asked the other staff working beside me what made them work in the lab every day—and they said, "I know I make a difference in someone's life every day, and that makes me feel good."

She listened, and then I asked her, "What made you work in a lab?" She thought for a few minutes and said, "It's the staff—my best friend works here."

And in retrospect, I knew 10 days ago that there was a difference on a Monday morning when there was chatter, bantering, kidding, and laughing as staff shared what they did with each other over the past weekend.

I honestly cannot thank you enough for sharing those books.

—Diane McClurg

We are fortunate to live in times in which there are great resources as well as great understanding of the importance of self-care. Today, creating a culture of well-being is not a nice thing to have, but a must-have. It is a necessary part of fulfilling an organization's mission. Yet even with this knowledge, the reluctance to be assertive in addressing well-being, stress, and trauma exists. The methods and tools above will change that. How we look at and address this important topic must be rewired. Prioritizing employee well-being can revitalize cultures and change lives.

CHAPTER 9

# Rewiring Retention

We have covered key aspects of rewiring retention throughout this book. The topic connects to the Human Capital Ecosystem™, selection and onboarding, and skill and career development. We are in retention mode even in the recruitment and selection process. The questions asked in those early check-ins—"Is this job what you thought it would be?"; "How can we make sure you feel supported?"; "I want you to feel safe sharing any concerns you have; how can I help with that?"—all build retention. So does getting to know someone's life outside of work. Each day we can build an employee's emotional bank account. When we hold the "battery charge" conversation and ask people, "Why are you in healthcare?" and, "Why here?" we are making retention deposits.

The laser-like use of data helps build retention. Employee engagement survey results provide ways to proactively reinforce what is working and adjust items that can be better. It also supports the personal development of each person. Engagement data shows skill and career building are strong needs for all the workforce in all roles. It provides the avenue to individualize development. Exit interviews are also helpful. Why did the person leave? Can adjustments be made to prevent others from departing? Are there patterns in the departures?

Another rewire is to re-interview those who are staying in the organization. In the book *Switch: How to Change Things When Change Is Hard*, authors Chip Heath and Dan Heath recommend focusing on successes or "bright spots." This is a good way to put that principle into practice. Talk to those who stay with you and represent different lengths of service, different roles, and workforce diversity. Ask these employees to answer the questions you are asking those being interviewed. Explain that their responses will help the organization hire people who are more likely to stay. They will help crystalize what to listen for in the interview process.

While the title of this book is *Rewiring Excellence*, the essence of the content is how to create a place that attracts and retains talent. Financial sustainability follows talent, and talent follows place. Over the years, we have been very involved in, and personally replenished by, creating solutions to challenges. Precision Leader Development™ (PLD) and OSAR™ are two recent solutions. Another solution has been moving to fewer rounding questions. Having fewer questions frees up caregivers to connect with patients in a deeper way (rather than a transactional way), which helps them feel that their work has purpose and meaning. This allows them to uncover, discover, and recover *why* they are in healthcare: to be useful and helpful to others. The bond that holds organizations together is relationships. Yes, technology is helpful and has a place. The magic of healthcare is people helping people.

Digging deep in data can provide solutions. People stay in jobs they like. When a nurse quits, for the most part, the intention is not to quit nursing. It is to quit where they are working. What will they miss most? Their coworkers. This is why coworkers are a component in the Human Capital Ecosystem. Each person stays or leaves for their own reasons. Finding out what those reasons are is the key to retention. Katherine Meese, PhD, and I collaborated on writing *The Human Margin: Building the Foundations of Trust*, which will be available in March of 2024 through the American College of Healthcare Executives (ACHE). The book reveals some key factors in employee engagement. So does the information gained in the Models of Care Insight Study described on the HPSG website. (See https://healthcareplussg.com/models-of-care-insight-study/ for details.)

Yes, people want to have a role that connects to their skill set and interests. They want a good team to be a part of. They want a leader and organization they trust. However, today it takes more to create a place people can't fathom leaving. This means an organization where leaders communicate well, a place where they can share their ideas and concerns, a place where they have the needed resources to do their work, a place where good work is recognized, a place where they feel a sense of belonging.

While this entire book is about retention of talent, a new method to implement is the personal retention plan, or PRP. Like Precision Leader Development (PLD), the PRP connects to each person individually. We are currently working with a health system that has around 300 people who are new to leadership. The PRP is so helpful. First, it lets the person know that retaining them is important. Just having the tool builds retention success. The process then encompasses conversations like, "We want you to feel this is the place for you. What are some things that create that feeling of belonging for you?" If the person gives an answer like "communication" or "input," try to drill down to get the conversation as specific as possible. Clarity is important to achieving the desired outcome.

We like personality profiles. We recently completed the Management By Strengths (MBS) process with a large group of new leaders. The individuals found the information helpful. It shows them that the organization values them as a person. It helps build relationships.

Here is a brief overview of how the PRP works:

Step One: Identify what the person is looking for and values in a workplace.

Step Two: Ask, "What are some things that would cause you to question or wonder whether this is the place for you?"

Step Three: Build empathy and understanding. In a situation where a person is relatively new to leadership, share that it is normal to have lots of emotions. (The five-minute video I did on this topic is helpful. Scan the QR code or visit https://healthcareplussg.com/resources/books/rewiring-excellence/ to view it.)

The point is, the leader may be feeling emotions on the inside and not be aware they are normal. A good question to ask is, "In your role, what is your biggest worry or concern right now?" It is not unusual to hear statements such as, "I am afraid," or, "I will fail," or, "I will let people down," or, "I am not sure I have the skill it takes." All of these are common emotions. This is a good time to share the commitment to supporting the person, talk about well-being resources, and then move to step four.

Step Four: Say, "We are committed to your success and investing in skill-building resources for you." While these resources will not be in the PRP, this step moves them to Precision Leader Development and OSAR. It helps the person see that the scope is one that they can handle. It is understood that skill building takes time. Their anxiety is reducing, and you will hear things such as, "I have never experienced anything like this before."

Step Five: Build on the growing foundation of trust by sharing about *you,* the person's supervisor. You have done this along the way. Here, share again what works best for you and how to best work with you. Often a person will not want to bother their leader, so proactively share with the person that they are not a bother. The PRP includes areas for the supervisor as well as the individual to identify actions each person will be taking to support the retention plan.

The PRP, and everything we do to get employees to stay, ultimately creates a culture where the best and brightest want to be. We spend time on both recruitment and retention. The more effective we are in retention, the more selective we can be in recruitment.

# CHAPTER 10

# Summary

The goal of *Rewiring Excellence* is to share some learnings to help organizations achieve their desired outcomes. The foundation is to take a fresh look at many current operational practices as they relate to the Human Capital Ecosystem™ in each organization.

You may notice the word "simple" has not been used till now. Why? While a communicator may use the word *simple* to mean the action was broken into bite-size pieces to make implementation easier, the receiver often hears the meaning as *easy*. There are very few *easies* in leadership! The goal is to help people and organizations narrow the scope of activities utilizing a stair-step approach to implementation. Less=always=consistency=better outcomes. Narrowing the scope also leads to more repetitions. Experience leads to better efficiency and effectiveness.

Precision Leader Development™ also helps the organization audit all the resources currently available for skill building. Often, more resources were developed to achieve better outcomes. If not built on the right platform, some are not utilized well and some are just not that good. A good system with the OSAR™ is designed to put a quality feedback loop in place. This means when a leader uses a resource, this feedback loop rates its value to them. This helps an organization reduce the number of resources to the best ones. This builds consistency.

Another learning from this fresh-eyed approach to diagnose, design, and implement is how important a person's direct supervisor is to their development. A quick assessment is to ask leaders, including members of the C-suite, what skills their direct reports are focused on and how they are assisting them in building that skill. We have found that even the most seasoned leader benefits from skill development in those they lead. Yes, organizational development and human resource specialists are valuable in skill building. However, more is accomplished when a leader sees that this professional has resources and sees themselves as developers. We are all chief development officers.

A final learning is around the role of technology. While it can be very helpful, it can be overused at times. The question is, *What will help the leader be most effective?* Much of the time, technology falls into the helpful category. The key is that the technology leads to better outcomes. Does it build relationships or take away from them?

We are finding there are times when having a checklist with questions to ask and an electronic tablet to document the answers gets in the way of a relationship. It comes off to employees as, "The leader is doing this because they must, and I am just a 'check the box' in their life." I know this is not the intention. An organization sent out a note to the leaders that they were going to suspend the use of rounding software and they trusted the leaders to continue to round and document as they felt best. The only requirement was to send a note to their leader each week on what they learned. They waited for the pushback. It has been eight months now (at the time of this writing), and none has come. Again, those who find technology helpful should use it. It is also good to say "pause." Pause something and see what happens. If results don't get better, you can always unpause the tool. The win was that this change showed the managers they are trusted.

There is enough great technology that is helpful; however, everything does not have to include it. The idea is to look at what works and when and how. I receive text messages to remind me when my immunotherapy appointment is. This is helpful and reduces staff time with calls. The goal is not to have an "all or nothing" policy. It is to determine what is working, what is not, and how less can be done while achieving better results. When I meet with my oncologist, while he looks on the computer and uses it for information and teaching, he sits so nothing is between us. It builds a relationship.

That is what rewiring is about. It is about looking at the facts and making decisions based on what is provided. If people who are not achieving results insist on doing it their way, ask, "How is that working for you?" When they say, "Not very well," then suggest trying another way.

I have not felt like I have worked in years. Why? I feel so blessed to spend my days with people in healthcare. I am in awe of you. You work too hard and deal with so many challenges. The goal is to bring an easier way to achieve the desired outcomes. What are the outcomes? To help those in leadership, thus all in healthcare, feel joy. You work too hard not to.

You are invited to come to our HPSG website. There are resources there, many of which are free, that can help you and your organization get even better and have an even bigger positive impact on your patients, employees, and organization. Please keep in touch as we travel this road of making a difference.

—Quint Studer

# Endnotes

**Chapter 1**
1. Studer, Quint. *Hardwiring Excellence: Purpose, Worthwhile Work, Making a Difference.* Fire Starter Publishing, 2003.

**Chapter 3**
1. Studer, Quint. *Hardwiring Excellence: Purpose, Worthwhile Work, Making a Difference.* Fire Starter Publishing, 2003.

**Chapter 4**
1. Chau VM, Engeln JT, Axelrath S, Khatter SJ, Kwon R, Melton MA, Reinsvold MC, Staley VM, To J, Tanabe KJ, Wojcik R. Beyond the chief complaint: Our patients' worries. J Med Humanit. 2017 Dec;38(4):541-47.
2. https://www.hcahpsonline.org. Centers for Medicare & Medicaid Services, Baltimore, MD. August 4, 2023.

**Chapter 8**
1. Studer, Quint, and Katherine Meese. *The Human Margin: Building the Foundations of Trust.* Health Administration Press (ACHE), 2024.

# About the Authors

**Quint Studer, BSE, MSE**

Quint Studer is a lifelong student of leadership. He has a gift for translating complex strategies into doable behaviors that allow organizations to achieve long-term success.

Quint is the author of 15 books, beginning with his first title, *BusinessWeek* bestseller *Hardwiring Excellence*. While most of his books are geared to those working in healthcare, two of his general business books—*Results That Last* and *The Busy Leader's Handbook*—became *Wall Street Journal* bestsellers. In 2021, he released *The Calling: Why Healthcare Is So Special*, which is aimed at helping healthcare professionals keep their sense of passion and purpose high. In 2023, the book *Sundays with Quint*, a collection of his most popular leadership columns, was released.

His new book, *Rewiring Excellence: Hardwired to Rewired*, provides tools and techniques that are doable and that help employees and physicians experience joy in their work as well as enhance patients' and families' healthcare experiences. *The Human Margin: Building the Foundations of Trust*, written in partnership with Katherine A. Meese, PhD, is due for publication in March 2024 by Health Administration Press (ACHE).

In his most recent venture to serve healthcare, he founded Healthcare Plus Solutions Group (HPSG), along with longtime colleague Dan Collard. The mission of the organization is to have a positive impact on those who receive care and those who provide care. HPSG specializes in helping healthcare organizations to diagnose and treat their most urgent pain points in order to achieve and sustain results. For more information, please visit https://healthcareplussg.com/.

## Dan Collard

Dan Collard is a seasoned healthcare executive with more than 29 years of healthcare industry experience spanning operations, consulting, and technology start-ups. He is the cofounder of Healthcare Plus Solutions Group, along with longtime colleague Quint Studer.

Most recently, Dan served as executive vice president and chief growth officer of TeamHealth, one of the nation's largest hospital-based physician practices. Prior to TeamHealth, Dan served as president of Press Ganey's Strategic Consulting Division and as CEO of EVOQ Medical, Inc., a healthcare technology start-up in Atlanta.

Dan spent 13 years at Studer Group® as a senior leader, where he served organizations ranging from rural hospitals to national health systems and academic medical centers. Prior to his time at Studer Group, Collard was a health system operator within LifePoint Health.

## ABOUT THE AUTHORS

Dan has always enjoyed the role of change agent within each organization he has led. In healthcare operations, Dan and his leadership teams helped their organizations attain best-in-class performance across a balanced set of metrics: quality, patient experience, physician and employee engagement, volume growth, and financial performance.

His passion for improving healthcare led to Dan's being asked to testify in June 2014 before the House Committee on Veterans' Affairs in the run-up to the bill signed into law that August.

# About Healthcare Plus Solutions Group

Healthcare Plus Solutions Group (HPSG) was founded by Quint Studer and Dan Collard in 2022 in Pensacola, Florida. Powered by a team of healthcare industry and talent management experts, HPSG specializes in delivering Precision Leader Development™ solutions to healthcare organizations across the continuum of care and their teams. With tightly customized services that look at the whole health of an organization, HPSG works closely with its partners to diagnose their most urgent pain points; design smart, collaborative solutions; and create a plan to execute in a way that delivers measurable results. With partnerships across the country, HPSG's primary mission is to have a positive impact on those who receive care and those who provide care. For more information, visit www.healthcareplussg.com.

# Other Books from Quint Studer

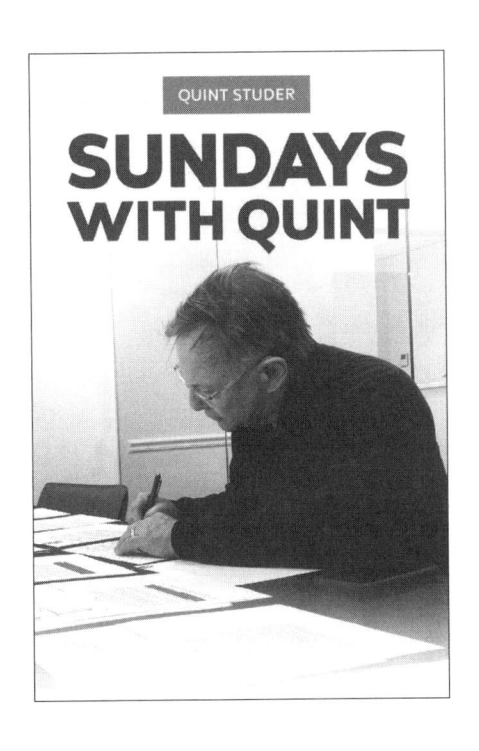

Each week, Quint Studer writes a popular leadership column for the *Pensacola News Journal*. This book shares 52 of these columns, each carefully curated for leaders, employees, and business owners in all industries. *Sundays with Quint* is meant for anyone wishing to benefit from the author's wealth of experience and his gift for breaking complex ideas into easy-to-grasp tips and tactics.

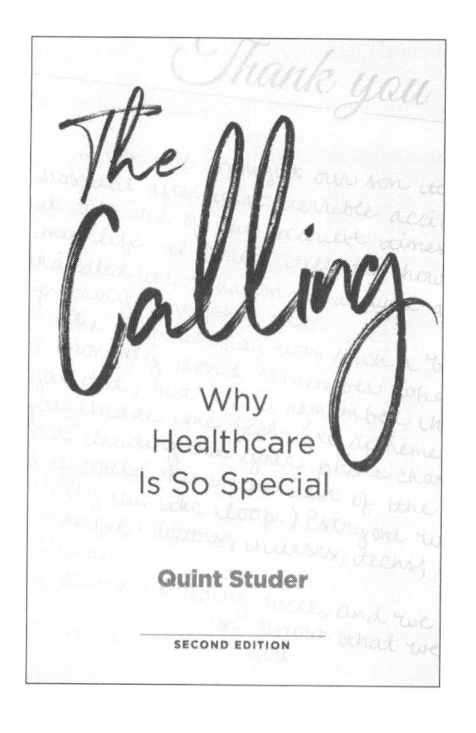

If there's one thing all healthcare people have in common, it's a great desire to be useful and helpful. This is our "calling," and we are born with it inside us. We enter the profession with a full emotional bank account. The challenge is to keep our sense of passion and purpose high so we can fully engage in the work we feel called to do.

In his book *The Calling: Why Healthcare Is So Special*, Quint Studer has pulled together a lifetime's worth of stories and insights designed to keep that emotional bank account overflowing—or to refill it for those who are running on empty.

The book is for anyone and everyone who works in healthcare and wants to keep their sense of calling alive. Written in the simple, practical, easy-to-process style that has become Studer's trademark—and packed with heartfelt stories that showcase the many gifts of healthcare people—the book will inspire clinicians and non-clinicians alike to become even more helpful and useful to those they serve.

---

**To order books, please visit**
https://healthcareplussg.com/resources/books

**To place a bulk order or for more information,** contact our team at info@HealthcarePlusSG.com.